Nursing Acceleration Challenge Exam (ACE) I PN-RN: Foundations of Nursing
Practice Questions

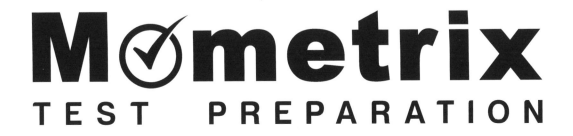

Dear Future Exam Success Story:

First of all, **THANK YOU** for purchasing Mometrix study materials!

Second, congratulations! You are one of the few determined test-takers who are committed to doing whatever it takes to excel on your exam. **You have come to the right place.** We developed these practice tests with one goal in mind: to deliver you the best possible approximation of the questions you will see on test day.

Standardized testing is one of the biggest obstacles on your road to success, which only increases the importance of doing well in the high-pressure, high-stakes environment of test day. Your results on this test could have a significant impact on your future, and these practice tests will give you the repetitions you need to build your familiarity and confidence with the test content and format to help you achieve your full potential on test day.

Your success is our success

We would love to hear from you! If you would like to share the story of your exam success or if you have any questions or comments in regard to our products, please contact us at **800-673-8175** or **support@mometrix.com**.

Thanks again for your business and we wish you continued success!

Sincerely,
The Mometrix Test Preparation Team

TABLE OF CONTENTS

Practice Test #1

1. Which of the following is usually restricted for 12 to 24 hours before a cardiac stress test?

    a. Caffeine

    b. Alcohol.

    c. Beta-blockers.

    d. Aspirin.

2. If a patient is becoming very upset and escalating into anger, which of the following is the best response?

    a. "What is your problem?"

    b. "It's time to settle down, ok?"

    c. "Your behavior is inappropriate."

    d. "You seem very upset."

3. If a patient who suffered a combat-related amputation of the left arm states, "I stay at home most of the time because people think I'm a freak," the patient is likely experiencing a problem with

    a. body image.

    b. self-esteem.

    c. mobility.

    d. motivation.

4. If a nurse is opening a sterile pack, which of the following actions will contaminate the contents? Select all that apply

    a. Holding the contents below waist level.

    b. Placing the pack on a clean, dry surface.

    c. Reaching across the sterile field.

    d. Applying sterile gloves after opening the pack.

5. A patient is admitted to the emergency department with acute asthma exacerbation. Arterial blood gases show

- pH 7.28
- $PaCO_2$ 48 mm Hg.
- HCO_3 25 mEq/L.

Which of the following acid-base imbalances do these findings indicate?

    a. Respiratory acidosis.

    b. Respiratory alkalosis.

    c. Metabolic acidosis.

    d. Metabolic alkalosis.

6. Patients with android (apple-shaped) obesity have an increased risk of

    a. heart disease.

    b. cellulitis.

    c. varicose veins.

    d. diabetes mellitus.

7. A poorly controlled diabetic patient is experiencing polydipsia and polyuria and has dry mucous membranes, poor skin turgor, and serum glucose of 368. Which electrolyte imbalance is most likely to be present?

    a. Hyponatremia.
    b. Hypernatremia.
    c. Hypokalemia.
    d. Hyperkalemia.

8. Which of the following statements about nonverbal communication is correct?

    a. Avoiding eye contact is a sign of dishonesty.
    b. Patients who appear relaxed usually have little anxiety.
    c. Standing very close to another person is a sign of aggression.
    d. Meaning can vary according to cultural background.

9. If a nurse examines his own personal history, trying to recognize biases and prejudices, this is an example of

    a. cultural awareness.
    b. cultural knowledge.
    c. cultural skill.
    d. cultural encounter.

10. In the communication process, if the patient notices an antiseptic odor and asks the nurse what the smell is, the smell represents the

    a. channel.
    b. referent.
    c. message.
    d. environment.

11. The purpose of teaching patients diaphragmatic breathing is to

    a. help clear the upper airways of secretions.
    b. increase the volume of inspiration.
    c. increase the volume of expiration.
    d. prevent respiratory infections.

12. For what reasons are older adults at increased risk of pressure ulcers? Select all that apply.

    a. Decreased lean body mass.
    b. Thinning epidermis.
    c. Increased oil production from sebaceous glands.
    d. Loss of collagen fibers and skin elasticity.

13. A patient who identifies as a lacto-ovo vegetarian will eat

    a. plant-based foods only.
    b. all foods.
    c. plant-based foods, chicken, and fish.
    d. plant-based foods, eggs, and dairy products.

14. If a Muslim patient refuses meals because of the onset of Ramadan, the nurse should

    a. remind the patient that the ill do not need to fast.
    b. arrange for meals during nonfasting hours.
    c. urge the patient to reconsider.
    d. ask family members to intervene.

15. A patient in the preoperative area expresses fear of the scheduled surgery and anxiety about the outcomes. The nurse's response should be to

    a. reassure the patient that everything will be ok.
    b. notify the surgeon that the patient does not want the surgery.
    c. hold the patient's hand and practice relaxation exercises.
    d. give the patient detailed information about surgery and recovery.

16. Following administration of a medication, a patient becomes anxious and restless with increasing dyspnea, cyanosis, itching, hives, and edema of the face and hands. What initial emergent treatment does the nurse anticipate?

    a. Oxygen.
    b. Oral antihistamine.
    c. Epinephrine.
    d. Bradycardia.

17. When a limb has been splinted, the distal limb should be checked for (1) circulation, (2) sensation, and (3):

    a. pain
    b. constriction.
    c. bleeding.
    d. movement.

18. A patient is prescribed nebulizer treatments with 0.25 mg budesonide/2 mL twice daily for asthma. Following treatment, the nurse should advise the patient to

    a. rinse the mouth with water.
    b. deep breathe and cough.
    c. avoid drinking cold fluids for one hour.
    d. sit upright for 30 minutes.

19. If the nurse reflects on her experience caring for patients and tries to identify ways in which she can improve her performance, this is an example of

    a. inference.
    b. evaluation.
    c. self-regulation.
    d. analysis.

20. Which of the following religious groups are generally forbidden by their religion to drink any alcoholic beverages? Select all that apply.

    a. Latter Day Saints (Mormons).
    b. Jews.
    c. Catholics.
    d. Muslims.

21. When positioning a patient on the side to relieve coccygeal pressure, the patient should be placed in a

    a. 10° lateral position.
    b. 30° lateral position.
    c. 60° lateral position.
    d. 90° lateral position.

22. Which of the following vaccinations is recommended for adults 60 and older?

    a. Meningococcal.
    b. Hepatitis A.
    c. Hepatitis B.
    d. Herpes zoster.

23. When assisting a patient with range-of-motion exercises, which motions should be carried out on the forearm? Select all that apply.

    a. Supination.
    b. Pronation.
    c. Rotation.
    d. Extension.

24. An older patient is confused, and the nurse is concerned that the patient may try to climb out of bed. Which of the following nursing actions should be avoided?

    a. Moving the patient to a room in view of the nursing station.
    b. Using a patient bed alarm.
    c. Placing the patient in physical restraints.
    d. Having a sitter stay with the patient.

25. If a patient has a nasogastric (NG)tube in place for drainage, but the NG tube has been obstructed and nonfunctioning for eight hours, the patient is at risk for

    a. gastric rupture.
    b. aspiration.
    c. infection.
    d. hypervolemia.

26. Which of the following complementary therapies involves focusing attention to quiet the mind and relieve stress?

    a. Biofeedback.
    b. Imagery.
    c. Yoga.
    d. Meditation.

27. Which of the following types of hepatitis is primarily spread through the fecal-oral route?

    a. Hepatitis A.
    b. Hepatitis B.
    c. Hepatitis C.
    d. Hepatitis D.

28. If the nurse is assisting a patient with a sitz bath, the temperature of the water should be at

    a. 95° to 100° F (35° to 37.7° C).
    b. 100° to 105° F (37.7° to 40.5° C).
    c. 105° to 110° F (40.5° to 43.3° C).
    d. 110° to 115° F (43.3° to 46° C).

29. When performing the Heimlich maneuver on an adult, the nurse should stand behind the patient and place a grasped fist

    a. above the umbilicus
    b. below the umbilicus
    c. over the epigastrium.
    d. over the sternum.

30. The nurse is caring for a patient who is receiving 1000 mL of intravenous (IV) fluid over eight hours. If the IV was started at 8 a.m., at what time should 250 mL remain in the IV bag?

    a. 10 p.m.
    b. 12 noon.
    c. 2 p.m.
    d. 4 p.m.

31. If a patient exhibits spikes and falls of fever that vary but never returns to normal, this pattern of fever is

    a. remittent.
    b. relapsing.
    c. intermittent.
    d. sustained.

32. If a vial contains 10 mg of medication in 1.5 mL and the patient's medication order is for 15 mg, how many mL should the nurse administer?

    _____ mL.

33. Which of the following behaviors on the part of the nurse could help to build trust?

    a. Using terms of endearment, such as "honey."
    b. Telling the patient to trust the nursing staff.
    c. Promptly responding to the patient's requests.
    d. Addressing the patient by first name.

34. Which member of the healthcare team is responsible for obtaining informed consent and telling the patient about the risks and benefits of a surgery?

    a. Physician.
    b. Anesthesiologist.
    c. Nurse.
    d. Admissions clerk.

35. Patients who receive repeated transfusions, such as patients with sickle cell disease, are especially at risk for

    a. deep vein thrombosis.
    b. hemorrhage.
    c. electrolyte imbalance.
    d. hemochromatosis.

36. Following a gastrectomy, a patient experiences dumping syndrome. Which of the following should the patient be taught about managing the syndrome? Select all that apply.

    a. Eat three meals daily.
    b. Avoid fluids for 30 to 45 minutes before and after meals.
    c. Avoid concentrated sweets, such as sugar and honey.
    d. Decrease protein and fat intake.

37. In the postoperative period, a patient who is groggy and awakening from anesthesia complains of severe nausea. The first response of the nurse should be to

    a. turn the patient on one side.
    b. advise the patient to take deep breaths.
    c. check orders for an antiemetic.
    d. notify the physician.

38. When doing oropharyngeal suctioning of a patient with left-sided paralysis, the best position for suctioning is

    a. supine, lying flat.
    b. side lying on the left.
    c. semi-Fowler's or upright.
    d. side lying on the right.

39. If a patient develops fever, chills, abdominal cramps, nausea, and vomiting 24 hours after eating undercooked chicken, the most likely causative agent is

    a. Staphylococcus aureus.
    b. Salmonella typhimurium.
    c. Escherichia coli.
    d. Clostridium botulinum.

40. If the nurse must deliver medications to four patients, and computers for documentation are available at the nursing station and at the points of care, then the most efficient method of documenting is

    a. to document at the point of care after each administration.
    b. to document at the nursing station after all administrations.
    c. to document at the nursing station before all administrations.
    d. to administer all medications and then document at points of care.

41. If the nurse finds that a patient has thrown a lit cigarette into a bedside trash can, starting a small fire that is filling the room with smoke, the priority action for the nurse is to

    a. pull the fire alarm.
    b. close the door to prevent spread.
    c. rescue and remove the patient from the room.
    d. put out the fire with an extinguisher.

42. If a patient complains of headache and nausea, this type of information regarding symptoms that are not evident externally is considered

    a. subjective data.
    b. objective data.
    c. incomplete data.
    d. discrete data.

43. If a patient's abdominal wound dehisces and a partial evisceration of intestines occurs, the nurse should

    a. leave the wound open to the air.
    b. cover the wound with sterile plastic wrap.
    c. cover the wound with dry, sterile dressings.
    d. cover the wound with sterile, saline-soaked dressings/towels.

44. A patient that the nurse is caring for is receiving intravenous (IV) fluids. The nurse notes that the area around the IV insertion site is swollen, pale, and cool to the touch. The most likely reason is

    a. inflammation.
    b. infiltration.
    c. allergic reaction.
    d. thrombosis.

45. A patient who has a severe cough experiences small amounts of urinary incontinence during episodes of coughing. This type of incontinence is characterized as

    a. urge incontinence.
    b. overflow incontinence.
    c. stress incontinence.
    d. functional incontinence.

46. If using the SOAP method of documentation, in which section would a patient's complaint of having a headache be documented?

    a. Subjective.
    b. Objective.
    c. Assessment.
    d. Plan.

47. In the *working* phase of a therapeutic relationship, who is responsible for health decisions and actions?

    a. Nurse.
    b. Patient.
    c. Physician.
    d. Family/Caregiver.

48. If the nurse has inserted a nasotracheal catheter for suctioning of a patient and the patient begins gagging, the nurse should

    a. apply suction while inserting the catheter.
    b. withdraw the catheter 2 to 3 cm.
    c. insert the catheter 2 to 3 cm more.
    d. remove the catheter.

49. Which of the following is a long, double-lumen tube inserted into the small intestine for drainage and decompression?

    a. Salem sump.
    b. Miller-Abbott.
    c. Cantor.
    d. Levin.

50. What actions should the nurse take when communicating with a hearing-impaired patient who wears hearing aids? Select all that apply.

    a. Stand in a position that allows the nurse to be seen, or touch the patient before speaking.
    b. Decrease background noises, such as the television.
    c. Speak in a normal tone of voice.
    d. Speak very slowly, and carefully articulate words.

51. When assisting a patient with bowel training to control fecal incontinence, which of the following stimulation methods should be avoided as much as possible?

    a. Digital stimulation.
    b. Mini enema.
    c. Enema.
    d. Suppository.

52. If a patient's pulse is thready and irregular, the best site for assessment is

    a. carotid.
    b. apical.
    c. temporal.
    d. radial.

53. Which of the following wound care products is most effective for a full-thickness ulcer (stage 4) that has heavy exudate?

    a. Alginate.
    b. Hydrogel.
    c. Hydrocolloid.
    d. Gauze dressing.

54. If a patient has experienced a stroke on the left side of the brain, he may exhibit

    a. left-sided weakness.
    b. impaired judgment.
    c. short attention span.
    d. impaired speech.

55. Patients who are lactose intolerant should avoid

    a. gluten.
    b. milk products.
    c. nightshade vegetables.
    d. soy products.

56. If a patient takes two to three abnormally shallow breaths followed by irregular periods of apnea, the breathing pattern is consistent with

    a. Biot's respirations.
    b. Kussmaul respirations.
    c. Cheyne-Stokes respirations.
    d. bradypnea.

57. Which of the following physical actions indicate active involvement in communication with a patient? Select all that apply.

    a. Standing beside the patient.
    b. Leaning toward the patient.
    c. Nodding the head.
    d. Maintaining eye contact.

58. Which of the following may result in a false low blood pressure reading?

    a. Cuff inflates too slowly.
    b. Arm is below the heart level.
    c. Cuff is too narrow.
    d. Cuff is too wide.

59. If nurse B, who is not assigned to a patient, asks to borrow nurse A's password so that nurse B can read the patient's electronic health record, nurse A should

    a. advise nurse B that the request is a HIPAA violation.
    b. provide the password to nurse B.
    c. suggest that nurse B ask the supervisor for permission.
    d. allow nurse B to read the record over nurse A's shoulder.

60. Which of the following complications is most common with ulcerative colitis?

    a. Fistulas.
    b. Anal abscess.
    c. Perforation.
    d. Strictures.

61. In order to comply with National Patient Safety Goals, before administering a treatment to a patient, the nurse must

    a. ask for an ID if not recognizing the patient.
    b. verify two forms of identification.
    c. verify the correct room and bed number.
    d. say the patient's name out loud.

62. If a patient is making statements that seem to be based on delusional thinking, such as "The doctor is constantly flirting with me," the best way to express doubt is

    a. "I don't believe that."
    b. "You must be kidding!"
    c. "Are you telling me the truth?"
    d. "That's hard to believe."

63. If a patient in an air-fluidized bed requires cardiopulmonary resuscitation (CPR), the nurse should

    a. turn off the bed's motor.
    b. remove the patient from the bed.
    c. position the patient on a backboard.
    d. proceed with CPR.

64. If using the SBAR method to organize information when communicating with a physician to report that a patient's condition is deteriorating, this information would be part of

    a. situation.
    b. background.
    c. assessment.
    d. recommendations/requests.

65. Which dietary restriction is especially important for patients with cirrhosis of the liver and severe ascites?

    a. Calcium.
    b. Sodium.
    c. Potassium.
    d. Magnesium.

66. When discussing diet with a patient, which of the following can the nurse use as an example of an incomplete protein?

    a. Legumes.
    b. Eggs.
    c. Milk/Milk products.
    d. Seafood.

67. The infectious disease that requires airborne precautions is

    a. influenza.
    b. wound infection (methicillin-resistant *Staphylococcus aureus* [MRSA]).
    c. *Bordetella* pertussis.
    d. tuberculosis.

68. If an older patient who weighs 143 pounds is to have an intake of 1.2 mg per kg protein per day to promote healing of a wound, how many milligrams of protein should the patient's diet include each day?

    _____ mg.

69. For which of the following types of urinary incontinence may Kegel (pelvic floor) exercises provide some control of incontinence? Select all that apply.

    a. Reflex.
    b. Functional
    c. Urge.
    d. Stress.

70. The factor that usually has the most influence on a patient's health is

    a. socioeconomic status.
    b. behavior.
    c. medical care.
    d. family history.

71. At which degree of angle should an intramuscular injection be administered in the deltoid muscle?

    a. 90°.
    b. 60°.
    c. 45°.
    d. 30°.

72. Which of the following is the most significant factor in determining if a patient with depression is at risk of suicide?

    a. Long-term history of depression.
    b. Low socioeconomic status.
    c. Previous suicide attempts.
    d. Lack of family support system.

73. If the nurse is ambulating with a patient and the patient starts to fall, the first action of the nurse should be to

    a. try to cushion the fall.
    b. grasp the patient's hands.
    c. grasp one of the patient's arms.
    d. place arms about patient's waist or grab the gait belt.

74. If a patient who is in alcohol recovery states, "I need a drink," the best response is

    a. "That sounds serious. Are you thinking about drinking?"
    b. "Just keep practicing your 12 steps."
    c. "Are you still attending your AA meetings?"
    d. "That's normal. Just try to think about your family."

75. If the patient's health record is organized as a *source record*, the nurse would expect

    a. all disciplines to document in the same section.
    b. each discipline to document in a different section.
    c. all documentation is done at a central location.
    d. all documentation must be completed at the point of care.

76. A rash with lesions that are less than 1 cm in diameter but circumscribed, solid, and slightly elevated is classified as

    a. macular
    b. vesicular.
    c. nodular.
    d. papular.

77. The nurse has collected a stool specimen for suspected *Clostridium difficile* infection but cannot transport it to the laboratory for testing for two hours. The nurse should

    a. store the specimen at room temperature.
    b. store the specimen in the freezer.
    c. store the specimen in the refrigerator.
    d. discard the specimen and obtain another one later.

78. Which of the following strategies are appropriate when caring for a patient with a radioactive implant? Select all that apply.

    a. Plan and organize activities to minimize time spent in the room.
    b. Limit the patient's visitors to two hours at a time.
    c. Wear a dosimeter and appropriate protection.
    d. Tell the patient to avoid ringing the bell for assistance.

79. The primary requirement for a patient to be treated under hospice care is that the patient

    a. has a life-threatening disease.
    b. has a life expectancy of six months or fewer.
    c. requires palliative care.
    d. has severe, unremitting pain.

80. If a patient has an ileostomy, which of the following foods should be avoided because of the risk of obstruction?

    a. Cheese.
    b. Asparagus.
    c. Onions.
    d. Raisins.

81. How long should the nurse auscultate for bowel sounds before determining that the bowel sounds are absent?

    a. 3 to 5 minutes.
    b. 2 to 3 minutes.
    c. 1 to 2 minutes.
    d. 30 to 60 seconds.

82. Side rails are not considered a restraint

    a. under any circumstances.
    b. unless the patient is confused.
    c. if only the top rails are elevated.
    d. if the bed is in the low position.

83. Which generation is most likely to want to receive health information electronically?

    a. Veterans (pre-1945).
    b. Generation X (1961 to 1980).
    c. Baby boomers (1945 to 1960).
    d. Millennials (1981 to 2000).

84. Following a generalized clonic-tonic (grand mal) seizure, a patient with epilepsy appears quite sleepy and exhibits muscle flaccidity, increased salivation, and confusion. The nurse should

    a. call for emergency assistance.
    b. allow the patient to rest until the postictal state passes.
    c. talk to the patient to encourage him to interact and rouse.
    d. sit the patient in an upright position.

85. A patient who has been sitting for a prolonged period stands up, takes a step, and then loses consciousness, falling to the floor in a faint that lasts for a few seconds. The nurse suspects

    a. postural hypotension.
    b. vasovagal reaction.
    c. slight stroke.
    d. cardiac abnormality.

86. The earliest indication of inadequate oxygenation is often

    a. cyanosis.
    b. confusion.
    c. gasping for breath.
    d. restlessness and anxiety.

87. If a patient has been ordered preoperative sedation, but she has not yet discussed the surgery with the physician or signed the informed consent, then the nurse should

    a. hold the sedation until the informed consent is completed.
    b. administer the sedation as ordered.
    c. ask the supervisor for advice.
    d. ask the patient to sign the informed consent.

88. When using the Z-track method of intramuscular injection, how far should the skin and subcutaneous tissue be pulled?

    a. 0.5 to 1.0 cm.
    b. 1.0 to 2.0 cm.
    c. 2.5 to 3.5 cm.
    d. 3.5 to 4.5 cm.

89. A patient nearing death has developed noisy, gurgling respirations. The nurse's first action should be to

    a. slightly elevate the patient's head.
    b. suction the patient's mouth and throat.
    c. request an order for an anticholinergic.
    d. take no action.

90. A patient was recently diagnosed with diabetes mellitus, type 1, and is very stressed about handling the disease. Which of the following is an example of an emotion-focused coping strategy?

    a. Working with a nutritionist.
    b. Attending diabetes education classes.
    c. Reading about the disease.
    d. Discussing fears and anxiety with the nurse.

91. If a patient is unable to swallow a capsule that contains beaded medication, the nurse should
   a. sprinkle the contents of the capsule over a dish of pudding or ice cream.
   b. open the capsule, crush the contents, and place in a measured volume of syrup.
   c. empty the capsule into a small measured volume of syrup.
   d. empty the capsule into a teaspoon and administer dry.

92. When communicating with an older adult with chronic illness, the nurse should
   a. treat the patient as a competent adult.
   b. make decisions for the patient.
   c. avoid worrying the patient about minor matters.
   d. discuss the patient's condition with the family instead of the patient.

93. In the chain of infection, the source of microorganisms is the
   a. etiologic agent.
   b. reservoir.
   c. vector.
   d. vehicle.

94. If a patient frequently climbs out of bed at night to go to the bathroom, the best solution is likely
   a. bedside commode.
   b. chemical restraints.
   c. physical restraints.
   d. scheduled toileting.

95. In the immediate postoperative period after extubation, which of the following respiratory rates should be reported to the physician?
   a. 8 per minute.
   b. 24 per minute.
   c. 12 per minute.
   d. 30 per minute.

96. If a patient tells the nurse, "The doctor has put a camera in my room to watch everything that I do," what type of delusion is she experiencing?
   a. Delusion of reference.
   b. Delusion of control.
   c. Delusion of grandeur.
   d. Delusion of persecution.

97. The Braden scale is used to
   a. stage pressure ulcers.
   b. plan treatment of pressure ulcers.
   c. predict the risk of pressure ulcers.
   d. monitor healing of pressure ulcers.

98. A patient has been receiving digoxin 0.5 mg per day, but the nurse is concerned that the patient is exhibiting signs of digitoxicity. Which of the following may indicate digitoxicity? Select all that apply.

    a. Tachycardia.
    b. Colored or halo vision.
    c. Constipation.
    d. Confusion, seizures.

99. How many hours should most older adults (65 or older) sleep during the night?

    a. 3 to 5 hours.
    b. 7 to 8 hours.
    c. 9 to 10 hours.
    d. 11 to 12 hours.

100. When removing an artificial eye, the nurse's first action should be to

    a. exert pressure below the lower eyelid.
    b. retract the upper eyelid.
    c. retract the lower eyelid.
    d. ask the patient to look upward.

101. If a patient has cirrhosis of the liver and is prescribed medications, which of the following is likely to be most impaired?

    a. Absorption.
    b. Excretion.
    c. Distribution.
    d. Metabolism.

102. If the nurse experiences a needlestick injury after giving a patient an injection, his initial response should be to

    a. wash the wound with soap and water.
    b. manually express blood from the wound.
    c. apply pressure to the wound.
    d. report the incident to a supervisor.

103. One thousand grams is equivalent to one

    a. dekagram.
    b. decigram.
    c. hectogram.
    d. kilogram.

104. Which of the following are risk factors for sleep apnea? Select all that apply.

    a. Obesity.
    b. Age over 65.
    c. Smoking.
    d. Sedentary lifestyle.

105. If a prescription for a wafer calls for "buccal administration," the nurse should

    a. dissolve the wafer in water before administering orally.
    b. place the wafer against the mucous membranes of the cheek.
    c. place the wafer on top of the patient's tongue.
    d. place the wafer under the patient's tongue.

106. If a patient complains of insomnia but naps for two hours in the afternoon and dozes on and off during the evening, the best solution is probably to

    a. take a sleeping aid.
    b. exercise before bedtime.
    c. stay awake during the daytime.
    d. drink warm milk at bedtime.

107. If a patient is receiving heparin therapy, the activated partial thromboplastin time (aPTT) should generally range from

    a. 25 to 35 seconds.
    b. 45 to 70 seconds.
    c. 60 to 90 seconds.
    d. 90 to 100 seconds.

108. If a malignant tumor is categorized as stage 3, this generally means that that the tumor

    a. is localized to the original site.
    b. has grown and begun to spread to adjacent lymph nodes.
    c. has spread to distant organs.
    d. has spread regionally to adjacent lymph nodes and muscle.

109. If levothyroxine is prescribed at 125 micrograms, the equivalent dosage in milligrams is
_____ mg.

110. Approximately how many mL are in one tablespoon?

    a. 6.
    b. 10.
    c. 16.
    d. 21.

111. If a patient believes that insects are crawling all over her skin, what type of hallucination is she experiencing?

    a. Tactile.
    b. Gustatory.
    c. Visual.
    d. Auditory.

112. When counseling a 26-year-old sexually active HIV-positive male about safe sex practices, the nurse should recommend which of the following? Select all that apply.

    a. Masturbation/Mutual masturbation.
    b. Unprotected sex only with other HIV-positive individuals.
    c. Condom use.
    d. Sexual abstinence.

113. If a patient indicates on admission for surgery that she will accept no blood products, which religion should the nurse believe the patient practices?

    a. Amish.
    b. Latter-day Saints (Mormon).
    c. Seventh-day Adventist.
    d. Jehovah's Witness.

114. When administering a dosage of medication through a metered-dose inhaler (MDI), the dispenser should be held

    a. inside the lips.
    b. one inch in front of the lips.
    c. two inches in front of the lips.
    d. three inches in front of the lips.

115. A spontaneous pneumothorax with accumulation of air in the pleural space occurring with no external wound is categorized as a(n)

    a. closed pneumothorax.
    b. open pneumothorax.
    c. tension pneumothorax.
    d. hemothorax.

116. If a patient is to receive 1,000 mL of dextrose 5% in water (D5W) over five hours with a drop factor of 15 drops per milliliter, the flow rate should be

    _____ drops per minute.

117. If a patient criticizes another nurse, stating that the nurse "refuses to answer any of my questions," which of the following is the best response?

    a. "I'm sorry, the nurse is probably busy."
    b. "Let's see if I can help you."
    c. "The nurse is very competent and caring."
    d. "I'm sure you misunderstood."

118. If a patient receives regular insulin on a sliding scale four times a day, how long before the patient is scheduled for a meal should the insulin generally be administered?

    a. 5 minutes.
    b. 15 minutes.
    c. 30 minutes.
    d. 60 minutes.

119. If a digoxin order is for 0.25 mg, but the medication is provided in 0.125 mg tablets, how many tablets should the nurse administer?

    _____ tablets.

120. Following the death of a patient, the nurse's first step in postmortem care should be to

    a. confirm organ donation status.
    b. collect specimens as needed.
    c. ask the family if they want to help.
    d. tag the body.

121. If a nurse is to administer a medication intramuscularly (IM) to an adult, the site that is preferred is the

    a. vastus lateralis.
    b. ventrogluteal.
    c. dorsogluteal.
    d. deltoid.

122. A patient with diabetes mellitus, type 1, complains of increasing thirst and abdominal pain and exhibits tachycardia, orthostatic hypotension, and Kussmaul respirations. The point-of-care testing that should be carried out immediately is

    a. electrocardiogram (ECG).
    b. electroencephalogram (EEG).
    c. urine ketones.
    d. blood glucose.

123. Which of the following is an absolute contraindication for a 65-year-old man wanting a prescription for sildenafil (Viagra) for erectile dysfunction?

    a. Patient uses a nitroglycerin transdermal patch (TransDerm-Nitro).
    b. Patient has a history of diabetes mellitus, type 2.
    c. Patient is taking a beta-blocker.
    d. Patient has a history of Parkinson's disease.

124. When a patient is crutch walking, how far away from the side of the foot should the crutch be placed?

    a. 4 inches (10 cm).
    b. 6 inches. (15 cm).
    c. 8 inches (20 cm).
    d. 10 inches (25 cm).

125. If a patient has a chest tube in place and experiences a sudden decrease in drainage, the nurse's first action should be to

    a. check the drainage system for obstruction/kinking.
    b. carry out a complete respiratory assessment.
    c. take the patient's vital signs.
    d. report this to the physician.

126. When assisting a patient with a bed bath, the area of the body that should be washed last is the

    a. face.
    b. hands.
    c. feet.
    d. perineum.

127. Paralysis associated with Guillain-Barré syndrome is usually

    a. descending.
    b. ascending.
    c. right-sided.
    d. left-sided.

128. Patients should avoid using nasal spray decongestants, such as oxymetazoline (Afrin), for more than 10 days because of the risk of

    a. allergic response.
    b. nosebleeds.
    c. rebound congestion.
    d. masked infection.

129. If a patient is receiving oxygen therapy per nasal cannula, the maximum flow rate is

    a. 3 L/min.
    b. 5 L/min.
    c. 6 L/min.
    d. 8 L/min.

130. Which of the following classes of drugs is used for prophylaxis and long-term treatment of asthma?

    a. Leukotriene receptor antagonist, such as montelukast.
    b. Synthetic glucocorticoid, such as prednisone.
    c. Xanthine derivative, such as theophylline.
    d. Beta-adrenergic agonist, such as albuterol.

131. If a patient is to have ice packs applied intermittently to an ankle four times daily, the maximum duration each time should be

    a. 5 to 10 minutes.
    b. 10 to 20 minutes.
    c. 20 to 30 minutes.
    d. 30 to 45 minutes.

132. Which of the following oxygen delivery systems best controls the specific oxygen concentration?

    a. Nasal cannula.
    b. Venturi mask.
    c. Simple facemask.
    d. Oxymizer.

133. According to Freud's psychosocial development theory, which agency of the mind is responsible for all drives and operates on the pleasure principle?

    a. Id.
    b. Superego.
    c. Ego.
    d. Active ego.

134. A normal BMI is

    a. 16.5 to 18.4 kg/m3.
    b. 18.5 to 24.9 kg/m3.
    c. 25 to 29.9 kg/m3.
    d. 30 to 34.9 kg/m3.

135. Which of the following are characteristics of middle adulthood (about ages 40 to 60)? Select all that apply.

    a. Achieving career satisfaction.
    b. Narrowing social involvement.
    c. Reassessing priorities of life.
    d. Increasing muscle strength/stamina.

136. The most common cause of chronic obstructive pulmonary disease (COPD) is

    a. genetic factors.
    b. history of lower respiratory infections.
    c. history of smoking.
    d. history of allergies.

137. If a 17-year-old burn patient who is normally even-tempered becomes frustrated while undergoing a painful dressing change and throws a screaming tantrum, the defense mechanism that the patient is exhibiting is

    a. displacement.
    b. introjection.
    c. compensation.
    d. regression.

138. When irrigating or cleansing a wound, the most commonly used solution is

    a. water.
    b. normal saline.
    c. hydrogen peroxide.
    d. betadine.

139. According to Kübler-Ross, which stage of grief is a patient likely undergoing if the patient, who has been diagnosed with cancer, begins to pray daily and to attend church regularly?

    a. Denial.
    b. Anger.
    c. Bargaining.
    d. Acceptance.

140. If a patient is on the dysphagia pureed diet (level 1), which of the following foods should be avoided? Select all that apply.

    a. Orange juice with pulp.
    b. Thickened milk.
    c. Pureed strawberries.
    d. Cream of wheat.

141. A patient is who newly diagnosed with Parkinson's disease is overcome with anxiety and despair, constantly worrying about his ability to cope when his condition deteriorates in the future. The type of grief that the patient is experiencing is called

    a. delayed.
    b. anticipatory.
    c. resolution.
    d. maladaptive.

142. Organic material, such as blood and fecal material, should be cleansed from objects and surfaces prior to application of a disinfectant primarily to

    a. prevent inactivation of the disinfectant.
    b. prevent residue buildup.
    c. decrease the contact time needed.
    d. decrease the amount of disinfectant needed.

143. If the nurse plans to use a bladder scanner to assess a patient's residual urinary retention, the scan should be done within

    a. 1 to 2 minutes of urination.
    b. 5 to 10 minutes of urination.
    c. 10 to 15 minutes of urination.
    d. 15 to 30 minutes of urination.

144. When changing a patient's colostomy bag following surgery, the nurse notes that the stoma appears dark purple. The nurse should

    a. change the bag because this is normal.
    b. reevaluate the stoma in 15 minutes.
    c. massage the tissue around the stoma.
    d. notify the physician.

145. If a patient is to receive 3 mg of albuterol sulfate syrup four times daily and the syrup contains 2 mg per 5 mL, how many milliliters of syrup should the patient receive for each dose? Provide an answer to one decimal point.

    _____ mL.

146. If a patient engages in running for about 75 minutes per week, how many times per week should the patient engage in strength training?

    a. once.
    b. twice.
    c. three times.
    d. four times.

147. The nurse should avoid lifting heavy items that weigh more than

    a. 20 lb.
    b. 30 lb.
    c. 40 lb.
    d. 50 lb.

148. If a patient has frostbite of both hands, the most likely treatment is

    a. enclosing hands in warm towels.
    b. immersing hands in cold water.
    c. immersing hands in warm water.
    d. immersing hands in hot water.

149. When cleansing instruments that are contaminated with blood, the instruments should first be
    a. rinsed in cold water.
    b. washed in warm, soapy water.
    c. rinsed with normal saline.
    d. soaked in a disinfectant.

150. Which of the following are signs of immune thrombocytopenic purpura (ITP)? Select all that apply.
    a. petechia, ecchymosis.
    b. epistaxis.
    c. dyspnea.
    d. bradycardia.

151. If a patient experiences frequent ingrown toenails, the nurse suspects that the patient
    a. has poor hygiene.
    b. uses an incorrect nail-trimming technique.
    c. has poor vision.
    d. goes barefoot much of the time.

152. What percentage of the body water is located in the intracellular space?
    a. 33%.
    b. 50%.
    c. 66%.
    d. 75%.

153. Which electrolytes are most prevalent in extracellular fluid (ECF)?
    a. Sodium and chloride.
    b. Sodium and potassium.
    c. Potassium and phosphate.
    d. Potassium and chloride.

154. Frequent contact with which of the following may most increase the risk of developing an allergic response?
    a. alcohol.
    b. latex.
    c. iodine.
    d. plastic.

155. Cobalamin (vitamin B_{12}) is not absorbed with
    a. iron-deficiency anemia.
    b. hemolytic anemia.
    c. aplastic anemia.
    d. pernicious anemia.

156. If a patient with chronic obstructive pulmonary disease (COPD) has been eating poorly because eating exhausts her, she should be advised to

 a. eat the largest meal in the morning.
 b. switch to pureed or liquid foods.
 c. rest for 30 minutes before meals.
 d. rest every 5 minutes while eating.

157. The movement of molecules from an area of high concentration to one of low concentration is referred to as

 a. osmosis.
 b. diffusion.
 c. active transport.
 d. fluid spacing.

158. When speaking with the spouse of a patient from Latin America, the nurse feels uncomfortable because the spouse stands very close when talking to him. The most likely reason is that the patient's spouse is exhibiting

 a. a cultural pattern.
 b. aggression.
 c. anger.
 d. insecurity.

159. If an electrical fire erupts on the unit, the fire extinguisher that is used must be labeled for which type of fire?

 a. Class A.
 b. Class B.
 c. Class C.
 d. Class D.

160. A Chinese patient insists on keeping very warm despite the heat and avoids certain foods that she describes as "cold," even though they are, in fact, warm. The patient is probably

 a. trying to keep yin and yang in balance.
 b. having chills.
 c. experiencing anxiety because of illness.
 d. suffering from delusions.

161. With which sexually transmitted disease is the infected female usually asymptomatic in the initial stages?

 a. Gonorrhea.
 b. Syphilis.
 c. Hepatitis B.
 d. HIV/AIDS.

162. If a patient was diagnosed with body lice, he should be advised to

 a. dry clean all clothes and linens.
 b. discard all clothes and linens.
 c. wash all clothes and linens in cold water.
 d. wash all clothes and linens in hot (130° F) water.

163. If a patient is being treated for anorexia, a reasonable goal for weight gain each week is
    a. 0.5 to 1 pound.
    b. 1 to 2 pounds.
    c. 2 to 3 pounds.
    d. 4 to 5 pounds.

164. According to Maslow, which of the following characteristics are possessed by self-actualized individuals? Select all that apply.
    a. The individual has an appropriate perception of reality.
    b. The individual is able to concentrate on solving problems.
    c. The individual is rational rather than spontaneous.
    d. The individual conforms to expectations.

165. With sickle cell anemia, sickling episodes are most commonly caused by
    a. infection
    b. trauma.
    c. blood transfusions.
    d. hypertension.

166. Which of the following are common sensory effects of aging related to vision? Select all that apply.
    a. Increased farsightedness.
    b. Color vision more acute.
    c. Declining vision.
    d. Eye lens softened.

167. Which of the following serving of foods is the lowest in fiber content?
    a. Oatmeal, 1/2 cup.
    b. White bread, 1 slice.
    c. Black beans, 1/2 cup cooked.
    d. Popcorn, 3 cups.

168. If a patient is taking warfarin (Coumadin), which of the following foods should the patient avoid consuming in excess because of the vitamin K content?
    a. Citrus fruits.
    b. Grains.
    c. Green, leafy vegetables.
    d. Milk products.

169. Which of the following is an example of a primary prevention?
    a. BP screening.
    b. Employment purified protein derivative (PPD) skin test.
    c. Routine Pap smear.
    d. Smoking cessation.

170. With polycythemia vera, which blood cells are affected?

    a. Platelets only.
    b. All types of blood cells
    c. Red blood cells only.
    d. White blood cells only.

171. A patient with arthritis complains of bilateral tinnitus. Which of the patient's medications may be the cause?

    a. Aspirin.
    b. Metformin.
    c. Fexofenadine.
    d. Metoprolol.

172. The term for personal standards regarding what is right or wrong is

    a. bioethics.
    b. values.
    c. morality.
    d. bias.

173. The moral principle that decrees that the nurse should do no harm when providing care to a patient is

    a. veracity.
    b. fidelity.
    c. beneficence.
    d. nonmaleficence.

174. Which of the following safety measures are fall prevention efforts in the home that the nurse should recommend? Select all that apply.

    a. The patient should move to a home that is all on one level.
    b. Tripping hazards should be removed.
    c. Grab bars should be installed in bathrooms.
    d. Lighting should be improved.

175. If the nurse is bathing a patient and the patient repeatedly tells the nurse to stop touching her, failing to do so could be considered

    a. assault.
    b. battery.
    c. negligence.
    d. malpractice.

176. Nursing practice is governed by

    a. place of employment.
    b. federal law.
    c. professional nursing organizations.
    d. state nurse practice act.

177. If a patient weighs 136.4 pounds, how many kilograms does the patient weigh? _____ kg.

178. If a nurse is assigned to care for a patient and drops the Foley catheter on an unsterile surface before inserting it, resulting in a urinary tract infection and sepsis, this action would be classified as

    a. negligence.
    b. unprofessional conduct.
    c. malpractice.
    d. gross negligence.

179. Which of the following is a common finding with left-sided heart failure?

    a. Pitting peripheral edema.
    b. Paroxysmal nocturnal dyspnea.
    c. Ascites.
    d. Distended jugular veins.

180. If a nurse threatens a patient with restraints if the patient doesn't stop complaining, this could be considered

    a. negligence.
    b. false imprisonment.
    c. battery.
    d. assault.

181. If a patient has a left trochanteric pressure ulcer that is full thickness with exposed subcutaneous tissue and slough, the pressure ulcer would be classified as

    a. stage I.
    b. stage II.
    c. stage III.
    d. stage IV.

182. When applying warm compresses, the nurse recognizes that maximal vasodilation occurs within

    a. 10 to 15 minutes.
    b. 20 to 30 minutes.
    c. 45 to 60 minutes.
    d. 60 to 90 minutes.

183. If a patient's heart rate recorded over a week from Sunday to Saturday was 66, 62, 72, 70, 74, 64, and 60, what is the patient's median heart rate?

    _____ beats per minute.

184. If the goal for a patient is "Patient will have relief from pain," which of the following is an appropriate desired outcome?

    a. "Patient will express fewer verbal/nonverbal indications of pain."
    b. "Patient will be free of pain."
    c. "Patient will appear comfortable."
    d. "Patient will ask for pain medication less often."

Answers and Explanations

1. A: Caffeine is usually restricted for 12 to 24 hours before a cardiac stress test because it may interfere with the results. Patients should be cautioned to avoid coffee and tea as well as other foods and liquids (such as chocolate and cola drinks). Patients should also be advised to avoid taking over-the-counter (OTC) pain medications, especially nonsteroidal anti-inflammatory drugs (NSAIDs) because many (including Anacin and Excedrin) contain caffeine. Some prescriptions (including Cafergot and Fiorinal) also contain caffeine.

2. D: If a patient is becoming very upset and escalating into anger, the best response is "You seem very upset." This statement is observational and is not challenging the patient or asking for an explanation of behavior. The nurse should maintain a low, calm tone of voice and avoid any accusatory or threatening statements or actions because the goal is to help the patient to de-escalate. The nurse may give the patient two options to help remove him-/herself from the situation, such as "Do you want to go to your room or walk with me?"

3. A: If a patient who suffered a combat-related amputation of the left arm states, "I stay at home most of the time because people think I'm a freak," the patient is likely experiencing a problem with body image. This is common with patients who have experienced some type of mutilation or change in the body, including patients who have suffered burns or undergone a mastectomy. Patients feel their bodies are out of step with cultural ideals, and this may impact their self-esteem.

4. A and C: If the nurse is opening a sterile pack, the actions that will contaminate the contents include (A) holding the contents below waist level. Everything below waist level is considered contaminated, so the surface upon which the sterile pack is placed must be elevated, dry, and clean. Also, choice (C), reaching across a sterile field, contaminates the field. Hands should be washed before opening the pack, but sterile gloves are donned after the pack is opened because the outside of the pack is nonsterile.

5. A: If a patient is admitted to the emergency department with acute asthma exacerbation, and arterial gases show pH 7.28, $PaCO_2$ 48 mm Hg, and HCO_3 25 mEq/L, then the acid-base imbalance that the patient is exhibiting is respiratory acidosis. The patient is acidotic because the pH is lower than 7.35. The problem is respiratory because the $PaCO_2$ is greater than 45 mm Hg, indicating hypoxia. The HCO_3 remains within normal limits, meaning that the respiratory acidosis is uncompensated.

6. A: Patients with android (apple-shaped) obesity have an increased risk of a number of chronic diseases, including heart disease, diabetes mellitus, breast cancer, and endometrial cancer. The visceral fat results in decreased insulin sensitivity, hypertension, increased triglycerides, and decreased HDL ("good") cholesterol. Android obesity is a higher risk factor than gynoid (pear-shaped) obesity; android obesity also results in increased free fatty acids being released into the blood.

7. B: If a poorly controlled diabetic patient is experiencing polydipsia and polyuria and has dry mucous membranes, poor skin turgor, and serum glucose of 368, the electrolyte imbalance that is most likely to be present is hypernatremia (a sodium level greater than 145 mEq/L). In this case, the hypernatremia results from fluid volume deficits. When the serum glucose level is elevated, the serum is hypertonic, and this pulls fluid from the cells and into the intravascular space, where it is eliminated through the kidneys.

8. D: The statement about nonverbal communication that is correct is: Meaning can vary according to cultural background. Although some behaviors, such as manner of making eye contact, are considered the norm for Americans, in fact, in our increasingly multicultural society, the nurse can't make assumptions as to meaning. The nurse should learn as much as possible about cultural differences.

9. A: If a nurse examines his own personal history, trying to recognize biases and prejudices, this is an example of cultural awareness because he is making an effort to look inward. Cultural knowledge is an understanding of differences among different cultures. Cultural skill is the ability to use cultural knowledge to assess patients and plan for their care. Cultural encounters involve engaging with members of different cultural groups. Cultural desire is the motivation to learn from members of other cultural groups.

10. B: In the communication process, if the patient notices an antiseptic odor and asks the nurse what the smell is, the smell represents the referent, the motivating force for communication. In the healthcare environment, many things may serve as referents, including sounds, smells, sights, feelings, and sensations. In the communication process, it's important for the nurse to understand what prompted the communication in order to better meet the needs of the patient. For example, if a patient is upset, the solution often depends on the referent.

11. C: The purpose of teaching patients diaphragmatic breathing is to increase the volume of expiration. Patients are taught to relax and allow their abdomens to protrude on inspiration and then to tighten the abdominal muscles and pull them inward and upward while breathing out through pursed lips. Diaphragmatic breathing is taught to patients with chronic obstructive pulmonary disease (COPD) so that the diaphragm can provide a mechanical aid to help rid the lungs of trapped air.

12. A, B, and **D:** Older adults are at increased risk of pressure ulcers because they have decreased lean body mass, and the epidermis tends to thin with age. Additionally, there is decreased oil production from sebaceous glands, resulting in dryer and more friable skin. The skin also has fewer collagen fibers, resulting in a loss of elasticity. Older adults may be less sensitive to pressure discomfort, and impaired mobility may limit the patient's ability to shift weight or turn.

13. D: A patient who identifies as a lacto-ovo vegetarian will eat plant-based foods as well as eggs and dairy products. A pescatarian eats all of the foods of a lacto-ovo vegetarian as well as fish. A vegan, on the other hand, eats only plant-based foods. A lacto vegetarian eats plant-based foods and milk products. A flexitarian is essentially a lacto-ovo vegetarian that occasionally eats meat but whose primary sources of nutrition are plant based, eggs, and dairy products.

14. B: If a Muslim patient refuses meals because of the onset of Ramadan, the nurse should arrange for meals during nonfasting hours (before sunrise and after sunset). Even if food services are not available, some food can be stored for the patient, or family members can be allowed to bring special foods for the patient. Although Islam does not require that the ill, elderly, or young fast during Ramadan, many devout Muslims will still choose to fast, and this should be respected.

15. D: If a patient in the preoperative area expresses fear of the scheduled surgery and anxiety about the outcome, the response is for the nurse to give the patient detailed information about the surgery and recovery. Patients are often fearful because they don't really understand what is going to happen to them, often because they were stressed when discussing the procedure with the physician. The nurse should take the time to answer any questions that the patient has.

16. C: Following administration of a medication, if a patient become anxious and restless with increasing dyspnea, cyanosis, itching, hives, and edema of the face and hands, the initial emergent treatment is likely to be epinephrine (adrenaline) because these signs are consistent with anaphylaxis, a severe allergic response. Epinephrine is the only treatment that is effective and works rapidly. Other supportive treatments may include oxygen, mechanical ventilation, intravenous (IV) fluids, and corticosteroids. Without immediate treatment, the patient may die.

17. D: When a limb has been splinted, the distal limb (below the splint or case) should be checked for

- Circulation: The distal pulse and capillary refill time should be checked to ensure that circulation is adequate to oxygenate the limb. Impaired circulation can lead to gangrene.
- Sensation: The temperature of the distal limb should be assessed against the other limb. Any numbness, tingling, or burning should be reported.
- Movement: The patient should be able to freely move the digits on the affected limb.

18. A: If a patient is prescribed nebulizer treatments with 0.25 mg budesonide/2mL twice daily for asthma, the nurse should advise the patient to rinse the mouth with water following treatment because budesonide is a steroid. If budesonide remains in contact with the mucous membranes of the mouth, the patient is at risk for the development of oral candidiasis because budesonide may depress the normal bacterial flora in the mouth, allowing the fungus to grow and multiply rapidly.

19. C: If the nurse reflects on her experience caring for patients and tries to identify ways in which she can improve performance, this is an example of self-regulation. Self-regulation should be an ongoing process. Inference is looking at data and understanding the significance. Evaluation is looking at circumstances and data objectively to reach conclusions. Analysis involves looking at information in an open-minded manner, attempting to determine what options are available.

20. A and D: The religious groups that are generally forbidden to drink any alcoholic beverages include Latter Day Saints (Mormons) and Muslims, although individual members of these religions may not follow this prohibition. Jews and Catholics are not prohibited from drinking alcohol, and, in fact, wine is part of the Jewish and Catholic sacraments. Buddhists typically avoid alcohol, and Hindus tend to use alcohol for medicinal purposes. Sikhs avoid all intoxicants, including alcohol.

21. B: When positioning a patient on the side to relieve coccygeal pressure, the patient should be placed in a 30° lateral position. The patient is essentially tipped toward the side rather than positioned directly onto the side because this position can result in pressure to the trochanteric areas and the lateral malleoli. If patients require turning to prevent tissue deterioration, they should be placed on pressure-reducing surfaces, such as special mattresses.

22. D: Adults 60 and older should receive the herpes zoster (shingles) vaccination. The vaccination is recommended even for individuals who have already experienced a shingles infection because the vaccination may prevent further occurrences or reduce the severity of the infection. The vaccination also reduces the risk of developing shingles by 51% and post-herpetic syndrome by 63%. The protection, however, lasts only about five years.

23. A and B: When assisting a patient with range-of-motion exercises, the motions that should be carried out on the forearm are supination and pronation. With supination, the arm and hand are turned so that the palm faces upward. Supination ranges from 70° to 90° and involves primarily the supinator and biceps brachii muscles. With pronation, the forearm is turned so that the palm faces downward. Pronation also ranges from 70° to 90°, and it involves primarily the pronator teres and pronator quadratus muscles.

24. C: If an older patient is confused and the nurse is concerned that the patient may try to climb out of bed, the nursing action that should be avoided is placing the patient in physical restraints because these restraints may increase the patient's anxiety. A patient bed alarm may be used to signal if the patient tries to get out of bed, or a sitter may stay with the patient. If possible, when patients are confused, they should be moved to a room in view of the nursing station.

25. B: If a patient has a nasogastric (NG) tube in place for drainage but it has been obstructed and nonfunctioning for eight hours, the patient is at risk for aspiration. This type of aspiration is often referred to as "silent" aspiration because the patient may not cough or show other indications that the gastric fluids are flowing into the lungs until the problem is severe. Because gastric fluids tend to be very acidic, they can burn the mucous membranes and lung tissues and cause severe inflammation.

26. D: Meditation is a complementary therapy that involves focusing attention to quiet the mind and relieve stress. Some people may concentrate on one word or phrase over and over again to prevent the mind from wandering. Others may repeat a mantra. The aim is to free the mind of all conscious thoughts as a healing method for the mind and body. Some people participate in religious meditation using items such as prayer beads and rosaries.

27. A: Hepatitis A is primarily spread through the fecal-oral route. Hepatitis A has an incubation period of 15 to 50 (average 28) days, and patients are most infectious during the two-week period prior to the onset of symptoms and remain infectious for another one or two weeks. Hepatitis A is associated with crowded conditions and poor personal hygiene and sanitation. Shellfish can become contaminated if they are in waters that contain fecal material. Infected food handlers often spread the disease. It can also be spread through sexual contact.

28. C: If a nurse is assisting a patient with a sitz bath, the water temperature should be at 105° to 110° F (40.5° to 43.3° C) and should be verified with a thermometer to avoid burning the patient. With a sitz bath, usually only the perineal or buttocks area is submerged in the water in order to increase circulation to the area and improve healing. Sitz baths are taken for 15 to 20 minutes, by which time the water temperature has usually fallen.

29. D: When performing the Heimlich maneuver on an adult, the nurse should stand behind the patient and place a grasped fist over the patient's abdomen above the umbilicus. This is the area of the diaphragm. Then, using the strength of both arms, the nurse should make quick upward thrusts to force air upward so that the air pressure forces the foreign object that is blocking the patient's airway to move. The procedure may need to be repeated several times.

30. B: If the nurse is caring for a patient who is receiving 1000 mL of intravenous (IV) fluid over eight hours and the IV was started at 8 a.m., 250 mL should remain in the IV bag at 2 p.m. Because the IV fluid is to run in over the span of eight hours (1000/8), this is a rate of 125 mL per hour. Placing a time tape that shows the expected level in the IV bag at different times can help to easily monitor IV fluid intake.

31. A: If a patient exhibits spikes and falls of fever that vary but never return to normal, this pattern of fever is remittent. The fluctuation of temperature is usually 2 degrees centigrade or more. This pattern of fever is very common with infectious diseases and may persist for varying durations. Remittent fever is not indicative of any particular disease or infection, although it is typical of typhoid fever and infective endocarditis.

32. 2.25 mL. If a vial contains 10 mg of medication in 1.5 ml, and the patient's medication order is for 15 mg, then the nurse should administer 2.25 mL. Formula:

- Milligrams needed/milligrams available in dose × volume per dose = current dose.
- $15/20 \times 1.5 = 1.5 \times 1.5 = 2.25$ mL.

33. C: Promptly responding to the patient's requests is a behavior on the part of the nurse that could help to build trust. This includes answering the patient's call bell as quickly as possible and taking time to respond to the patient's questions. The nurse should avoid using terms of endearment, such as "honey," or addressing patients by their first names unless asked to do so. Telling the patient that the nursing staff can be trusted is not the same as demonstrating actions that build trust.

34. A: The member of the healthcare team that is responsible for obtaining informed consent and telling the patient about the risks and benefits of a surgery is the physician, even though other team members may actually witness and sign the informed consent form. Informed consent should include an explanation of the diagnosis, nature and reason for the procedure, alternative options, and risks and benefits of having the procedure and of not having the procedure.

35. D: Patients who receive repeated transfusions, such as patients with sickle cell disease, are especially at risk for hemochromatosis (iron overload). Patients are at risk if they have had more than eight transfusions. Because this type of iron overload is secondary and the transfusions are provided because of anemia, phlebotomy is not usually an acceptable treatment because it may worsen the anemia, so patients must undergo chelation therapy, such as with deferiprone or deferasirox, to remove the excess iron.

36. B and C: If a patient experiences dumping syndrome following a gastrectomy, the patient should be taught to avoid fluids for 30 to 45 minutes before and after meals because of the reduced capacity. Patients should eat six small meals daily rather than three large meals and should avoid concentrated sweets, such as sugar and honey because these may cause diarrhea and dizziness. Patients may need to increase protein and fat intake to ensure adequate nutrition and recovery.

37. A: In the postoperative period, if a patient who is groggy and awakening from anesthesia complains of severe nausea (or any degree of nausea), the first response of the nurse should be to turn the patient on one side. If the patient remains supine and vomits, the patient may easily aspirate or even asphyxiate, resulting in death. On the side, the vomitus may drain out of the mouth more easily. The patient should receive an antiemetic if the nausea persists.

38. C: When doing oropharyngeal suctioning of a patient with left-sided paralysis, the best position for suctioning is semi-Fowler's or upright with the patient lying supine because this position gives good visualization and access for the nurse. The Yankauer suction device (tonsillar tip) is used for oropharyngeal suctioning because it has a large, rigid tip with both large and small openings and is angled to fit easily into the mouth to suction mucus.

39. B: If a patient develops fever, chills, abdominal cramps, nausea, and vomiting 24 hours after eating undercooked chicken, the most likely causative agent is *Salmonella typhimurium*. Salmonellosis may also develop from other undercooked meats and raw eggs. Infection is more likely to occur in the summer than winter, and children, the elderly, and the immunocompromised are most at risk. People who handle reptiles, small rodents, and baby chicks may carry *S. typhimurium* on their hands and pass it onto food if they don't wash their hands adequately.

40. D: If the nurse must deliver medications to four patients, and computers for documentation are available at the nursing station and at the point of care, the most efficient method of documenting is to document at the point of care after each administration. Documentation should always be done promptly and not put off until a later time. The nurse should never document in advance in anticipation of carrying out a procedure but only after completion.

41. C: If the nurse finds that a small fire is filling a patient's room with smoke, the priority action for the nurse is to rescue and remove the patient, although the nurse should certainly call for help while doing so. According to the RACE process, the steps to fire response include

- Rescue: The patient must always be secured first.
- Alarm: The fire alarm should be sounded.
- Contain: Doors and windows should be shut if this can be done safely.
- Extinguish: An attempt can be made to extinguish the fire with the nearest fire extinguisher if it is safe to do so.

42. A: If a patient complains of headache and nausea, this type of information regarding symptoms that are not evident externally is considered subjective data because they are based on a person's statement or opinions and cannot be verified through measure. Objective data are observable and measurable. For example, if a patient has a "red, raised papular rash," this information is objective. Objective data are stronger than subjective data, which may be open to interpretation, falsified, or mistaken.

43. D: If a patient's abdominal wound dehisces and a partial evisceration of intestines occurs, then the nurse should cover the wound with sterile saline-soaked dressings/towels. The purpose of soaking the dressings with saline is to prevent them from adhering to the eviscerated organs and damaging the tissue. Evisceration is a medical emergency, and the physician should be notified immediately and the patient should be prepared for a return to surgery. The eviscerated organs should be assessed for signs of ischemia. The patient should be maintained in the supine position with the knees slightly flexed.

44. B: If a patient the nurse is caring for is receiving intravenous fluids, and the nurse notes that the area around the IV insertion site is swollen, pale, and cool to the touch, then the most likely reason is that the needle has infiltrated and the IV solution is entering the tissue instead of the vein. The IV should be immediately clamped to prevent further tissue damage. The IV should be discontinued and restarted at another site.

45. C: If a patient who has a severe cough experiences small amounts of urinary incontinence during episodes of coughing, it is characterized as stress incontinence. Urine leakage occurs because of the sudden increase in intra-abdominal pressure, which can also occur with laughing, straining to carry or lift materials, bowling, jogging, playing tennis or golf, or sneezing. Patients should be instructed to use the "knack" method (quick tightening of the pelvic floor muscles) to help prevent incontinence.

46. A: If using the SOAP method of documentation, a patient's complaint of having a headache would be documented in the *subjective* section:

- Subjective: Patient's directly quoted description of problems.
- Objective: Nurse's observations and measurements.
- Assessment: Nursing diagnosis based on the subjective description and objective data.
- Plan: Plan of care to alleviate the problems.

32

Each separate SOAP note is numbered consecutively with interventions matched to the correct number. In some cases, an additional I and E (SOAPIER) are added for interventions and evaluation.

47. B: In the *working* phase of a therapeutic relationship, the person who is responsible for health decisions and actions is the patient. The working phase is preceded by the preinteraction phase and the orientation phase. During the working phase, the nurse provides support to the patient, who begins exploring and understanding feelings and thoughts and taking actions. The nurse develops feelings of empathy and caring toward the patient. The working phase is followed by the termination phase.

48. D: If the nurse has inserted a nasotracheal catheter for suctioning of a patient and the patient begins gagging, then the nurse should remove the catheter because it has likely entered the patient's esophagus. The catheter should be discarded and the procedure started again with a new catheter. The patient should be cautioned to avoid swallowing while the catheter is inserted, and no suctioning should take place during insertion. Insertion should be only on inhalation.

49. B: Miller-Abbott is a long, double-lumen tube inserted into the small intestine for drainage and decompression. The Salem sump tube is also a double-lumen tube, but it is short and contains a small vent tube within the larger tube to help reduce pressure at the distal end to less than 24 mm Hg in order to prevent tissue damage. The Cantor tube is a single-lumen tube that contains an inflatable balloon at the distal end to prevent the tube from migrating. The Levin tube is a single-lumen tube with a solid end.

50. A, B, and **C:** The actions that the nurse should take when communicating with a hearing-impaired patient who wears hearing aids include moving into the room and standing in a position that allows the nurse to be seen or to touch the patient before speaking to avoid startling the patient. The nurse should try to decrease background noises, such as the television, and should speak in a normal tone of voice, facing the patient in case the patient uses lip-reading assistance. It is not necessary to speak very slowly or to carefully articulate words.

51. C: When assisting a patient with bowel training to control fecal incontinence, the stimulation method that should be avoided as much as possible is the use of enemas, although small-volume mini enemas may be used to stimulate the anorectal reflex. Rectal suppositories, such as glycerin or bisacodyl, may be inserted 5 to 30 minutes before scheduled defecation. Digital stimulation with a gloved and lubricated finger inserted into the anal canal may stimulate and dilate the anal sphincter.

52. B: If a patient's pulse is thready and irregular, the best site for assessment is the apical pulse. Although any artery can be used to assess the pulse, the radial artery is most commonly used, but if blood pressure is low or the pulse is irregular, the radial count may be inaccurate. The bell side of a stethoscope should be used to assess the heart sounds because it better detects the low-pitched sounds of blood movement than does the diaphragm side. The bell should be applied lightly to the skin.

53. A: The wound care product that is most effective for a full-thickness ulcer (stage 4) that has heavy exudate is alginate. Alginates are derived from seaweed and are highly absorptive. Alginate transforms into a gel as it absorbs the exudate, helping to keep the exudate contained in the dressing. Alginates should not be used with third-degree burns, nondraining wounds, and dry necrotic wounds. Alginates should be loosely packed into a wound and layered for deep wounds. Dressings should be changed every 24 hours.

54. D: If a patient has experienced a stroke on the left side of the brain, he may exhibit impaired speech because this side of the brain contains the speech centers. Patients may experience different types of speech impairment:

- Wernicke's aphasia: This is receptive aphasia that results in impaired comprehension, and the person's speech often makes little sense.
- Broca's aphasia: This is expressive aphasia. Patients may have varying degrees of comprehension but much difficulty in responding.
- Global aphasia: This is the most severe aphasia and includes both receptive and expressive aphasia.

55. B: Patients who are lactose intolerant should avoid milk products. Patients with lactose intolerance lack the enzyme lactase, which is needed to properly digest the lactose in milk products. Because the lactose is not adequately digested, it results in increased production of gas and diarrhea. Live acidophilus culture added to the diet helps convert the lactose into a form of sugar that the body can digest. Patients may also take oral lactase (Lactaid) as a supplement with milk products.

56. C: If a patient takes two to three abnormally shallow breaths followed by irregular periods of apnea, the breathing pattern is consistent with Cheyne-Stokes respirations (aka periodic breathing). The cycle usually begins with slow, shallow breaths that increase in rate and depth, after which the breathing then slows again and ends in a period of apnea that persist for 10 to 20 seconds. Cheyne-Stokes respirations may occur with congestive heart failure and encephalitis as well as after a fast ascent to high elevations (altitude sickness), but this pattern is most commonly found with patients who are nearing death.

57. B, C, and **D:** Physical actions that indicate active involvement in communication with a patient include leaning slightly toward the patient when the patient is talking, nodding the head to indicate that the nurse is paying attention, and maintaining eye contact (as is appropriate culturally). The nurse should stand facing the patient instead of beside the patient because it is difficult for the patient to observe the reactions of the nurse to the side.

58. D: If a blood pressure cuff is too wide for the patient, this can result in a false low blood pressure reading. Other causes of low readings can include deflating the cuff too quickly (low systolic), placing the arm above the level of the heart, or incorrectly placing the stethoscope. If inflation is not adequate, a low reading may also occur. In contrast, false high readings may occur if the blood pressure cuff is too narrow or is wrapped too loosely about the arm. A false high reading can also occur if the arm is below the level of the heart or if the cuff is inflated too slowly.

59. A: If nurse B, who is not assigned to a patient, asks to borrow nurse A's password so that nurse B can read the patient's electronic health record, nurse A should advise nurse B that the request is a HIPAA violation of privacy and security. Under no circumstances should passwords be shared, and "shoulder surfing" — reading over another nurse's shoulder — is also a violation. Only healthcare professionals who have been granted access should read a patient's records, and then only to the extent necessary for the provision of care.

60. C: Perforation is a complication that is most common with ulcerative colitis. Fistulas and anal abscesses rarely occur, and strictures occur only occasionally. Other common complications include pseudopolyps, rectal bleeding, diarrhea, abdominal cramping, tenesmus, and toxic megacolon. The risk of carcinoma increases after 10 years of the disease. The usual age of onset is during adolescence and early adulthood.

34

61. B: In order to comply with the National Patient Safety Goals, before administering a treatment to a patient, the nurse must verify two forms of identification, even if the nurse recognizes the patient. If a patient is hospitalized, this usually means checking the patient's ID bracelet to confirm the right patient and to ask the patient's for his or her birthdate. The room and bed numbers should always be verified, but these alone are not considered adequate identification of a patient. Patients who are confused or hard of hearing may respond to an incorrect name.

62. D: If a patient is making statements that seem to be based on delusional thinking, the best way to express doubt is: "That's hard to believe." This statement is not overtly challenging, but it does avoid reinforcing false beliefs, and it may help to undermine the patient's faulty belief system. The nurse should avoid arguing with the patient or directly confronting the patient's false statements because this is rarely effective, but should remain calm and try to reset reality.

63. A: If a patient in an air-fluidized bed needs CPR, the nurse should turn off the bed's motor because this causes the bed surface to settle and firm. Air-fluidized beds pump air through tiny silicone-coated spheres contained in a frame, a process that results in a fluidlike surface, allowing the patient to essentially float. Air-fluidized beds are indicated for patient with large and/or multiple pressure ulcers (stages III and IV). Because the patient requires less frequent turning, shear and friction are reduced.

64. C: If using the SBAR method to organize information when communicating with a physician to report that a patient's condition is deteriorating, the information would be part of *assessment*:

- Situation: Statement of the problem.
- Background: Information that is pertinent to the problem.
- Assessment: Current findings, such as vital signs (VSs) and changes in condition.
- Recommendations/Requests: Need for treatment, tests, physician visit.

The SBAR method is also commonly used for hand-off communication, such as at the change of shift.

65. B: The dietary restriction that is especially important for patients with cirrhosis of the liver and severe ascites is sodium. The higher the intake of sodium, the more fluid is retained. Treatment for ascites also includes diuretics and fluid removal, although routine paracenteses are no longer done because the fluid almost immediately begins to reaccumulate and additional electrolytes are lost in the procedure. A peritoneovenous shunt may be done to continuously reinfuse the ascitic fluid back into circulation, although this surgery is not routinely done because of numerous possible complications.

66. A: When discussing diet with a patient, the nurse explains that an example of an incomplete protein is legumes (such as navy beans). Complete proteins contain all nine essential amino acids, whereas incomplete proteins lack some of these amino acids. Complete proteins are found primarily in animal-based proteins, such as those found in meats, eggs, and milk products. However, a few plant-based foods, such as quinoa and chia seeds, contain complete proteins. Incomplete proteins, such as those found in rice, beans, nuts, and whole grains, should be combined.

67. D: The infectious disease that requires airborne precautions is tuberculosis. Other diseases that require airborne precautions include severe acute respiratory syndrome (SARS), measles, and varicella (chickenpox). Hospitalized patients should be placed in negative pressure (airborne infection isolation rooms). Personal protective equipment (PPE) includes a fit-tested N95 or higher respirator and gloves, gown, and a face shield if the nurse may come in contact with respiratory fluids. Airborne pathogens may remain suspended in the air for several hours and can travel considerable distances in air currents.

68. 78 mg. If an older patient who weighs 143 pounds is to have an intake of 1.2 mg per kg protein per day to promote healing of a wound, the patient's diet should include 78 mg daily. The first step is to convert pounds to kilograms: 143 lb./2.2 = 65 kg. The next step is to multiply the desired milligrams by the number of kilograms: 65 × 1.2 = 78 mg.

69. C and D: Kegel (pelvic floor) exercises can provide some control of incontinence for urge and stress incontinence because both involve the lack of adequate sphincter control. Kegel exercises must be done 40 to 50 times a day in order to strengthen the muscles. Kegel exercises may also be used for patients with fecal incontinence. Pelvic floor muscle rehabilitation may also be done with vaginal weight training, biofeedback, and electrical stimulation.

70. B: The factor that usually has the most influence on a patient's health is the patient's behavior, including the lifestyle choices that the patient has made over the entire course of life, not just recent behavior. Behavioral choices that have a particularly negative effect on health include smoking, overeating, having poor nutrition and diet (fast food, high sodium, high fat), drinking alcohol to excess, and failing to exercise adequately. Other behavioral choices can include failing to get immunized, follow through with treatment, and take medications as prescribed.

71. A: An intramuscular injection should be administered into the deltoid and other muscles at a 90° angle. If the patient is very thin or the deltoid muscle is underdeveloped, then the ventrogluteal or other sites are preferred. It's important that the needle be vertical to the skin so that the medication is injected into the muscle and not into the subcutaneous tissue because that may cause irritation and problems with absorption.

72. C: The most significant factor in determining if a patient with depression is at risk of suicide is a previous suicide attempt. The patient must be asked directly if he is considering suicide and if he has made a plan to kill himself. Other risk factors include lack of support and current mental disorders as well as evidence of increasing substance abuse. Males are more likely to commit suicide than females. The nurse must remain calm, supportive, and nonjudgmental.

73. D: If the nurse is ambulating with a patient and the patient starts to fall, the first action of the nurse should be to place the arms around the patient's waist (from behind) or grab the gait belt. The nurse should stand with feet apart in order to provide a stable base and slide one leg forward against the patient so that the patient can slide against the leg with support onto the floor without falling. As the patient slides down, the nurse should bend the knees and lower the body.

74. A: If a patient who is in alcohol recovery states, "I need a drink," the best response is, "That sounds serious. Are you thinking about drinking?" This statement validates the patient's statement and gives the patient the opportunity to discuss the feelings that prompted the statement without changing the subject, expressing disapproval, and asking excessively probing questions. The nurse should be careful to avoid minimizing the patient's feelings or providing false reassurance.

75. B: If the patient's health record is organized as a *source record,* the nurse would expect each discipline to document in a different section. This is the traditional manner of organizing patient's records. However, with this type of record, finding information can be time consuming and inefficient because the healthcare provider must switch from one section to another to get the full picture. More modern records still use some aspects of the source record. For example, physician's notes are usually separate, whereas nursing, physical therapy (PT), and occupational therapy (OT) may be together.

76. D: A rash with lesions that are less than 1 cm in diameter but circumscribed, solid, and slightly elevated is classified as papular. If the lesions are more than 1 cm in size, they are classified as plaques. Nodules are similar to papules but extend deeper into the dermis so they may feel more solid. Vesicles are circular circumscribed lesions smaller than 0.5 cm and filled with fluid (serous fluid or blood). If the lesions are larger than 0.5 cm, they are classified as bullae. Macules are flat lesions with a change of color, such as a freckle.

77. C: If the nurse has collected a stool specimen for a suspected *Clostridium difficile* infection but cannot transfer it to the laboratory for testing for two hours, she should store the specimen in the refrigerator. Spores degrade rapidly at room temperature, so the results obtained in two hours may be completely compromised. Ideally, specimens should be immediately transported to the lab for testing. Tests for *C. difficile* include stool culture, polymerase chain reaction (PCR) assays, antigen detection, and toxin testing.

78. A and C: If a patient has a radioactive implant, it's important to limit time spent in the room, so the nurse should plan well and organize activities so that multiple tasks can be done while he is in the room in order to minimize time. The nurse should wear a dosimeter and appropriate protection according to guidelines provided by radiology. The patient should be aware of the time restrictions, but the patient should be assured that the nurse will respond if the patient rings the call bell. Visitors are limited to 30 minutes at a time.

79. B: The primary requirement for a patient to be treated under hospice care is that the patient has a life expectancy of fewer than six months. However, because determining life expectancy is an inexact science, hospice can be renewed if the patient continues to live past six months but death still appears reasonably imminent. Another primary requirement is that the patient undergo palliative care but not further curative treatments. Patients who are cared for under hospice can choose to opt out and seek further treatment.

80. D: If a patient has an ileostomy, foods that the patient may swallow whole or with minimal chewing, such as raisins, nuts, popcorn, raw vegetables, corn, and seeds, should be avoided because they may result in obstruction. Patients must also be advised about foods that are odor producing (eggs, fish, garlic, asparagus, cabbage, broccoli), gas forming (beans, cabbage, onions, carbonated drinks, sprouts, and strong cheeses), and diarrhea causing (alcoholic beverages, cabbage, spinach, green beans, spicy foods, raw fruits, and coffee).

81. A: The nurse should auscultate the bowel sounds for three to five minutes before determining that bowel sounds are absent. The nurse should listen carefully in all four quadrants of the abdomen, and it can take up to a minute to hear bowel sounds in each area. The nurse should use care to avoid massaging the abdomen or pressing too hard with the stethoscope when assessing for sounds. If bowel sounds are absent, the abdomen is often taut and distended.

82. C: Side rails are not considered a restraint if only the top rails are elevated because these are used as a safety measure to prevent the patient from falling out of bed and as a turning aid. If the lower rails are lowered, the patient can still swing to the side and sit up. However, if both sets of side rails are elevated, then this restrains the patient, and this means of restraint is often unsafe because patients may climb over the side rails and fall.

83. D: The generation that is most likely to want to receive health information electronically through emails, websites, and text messages is Millennials, who were born between 1981 and 2000. This generation has always known the computer and electronic equipment, and they are generally not intimidated by the digital world. Many carry out much of their communication through text messaging on smartphones. They often prefer information in small chunks.

84. B: Following a generalized clonic-tonic (grand mal) seizure, a patient with epilepsy who appears quite sleepy and exhibits muscle flaccidity, increased salivation, and confusion should be allowed to rest until the postictal state passes. This period usually lasts for a few minutes to a half hour, although it may persist for an hour if the seizure was severe. During the postictal period, the brain is recovering from the effects of the seizure.

85. A: If a patient who has been sitting for a prolonged period stands up, takes a step, and then loses consciousness, falling to the floor in a faint that lasts for a few seconds, the nurse should suspect postural hypotension. This can be verified by doing tilt table blood pressure testing or by taking a series of blood pressure measurements with the patient changing position from lying and sitting to determine if there is a significant drop in blood pressure.

86. D: The earliest indications of inadequate oxygenation are often restlessness and anxiety. The patient's skin and mucous membranes may appear pale. The patient may exhibit tachypnea and tachycardia and experience increasing dyspnea and hypertension. Patients may also complain of headache. As the condition worsens, the patient's blood pressure, pulse, and rate of respirations may begin to fall and cyanosis may be evident as well as cardiac dysrhythmias. Patients may become increasingly confused and stuporous.

87. B: If a patient has been ordered preoperative sedation, but the patient has not yet discussed the surgery with the physician or signed the informed consent, then the nurse should hold the sedation until the informed consent is completed because the patient should not be sedated before signing. It is the physician's responsibility to obtain informed consent, although the nurse can witness the signing of the consent form if the physician has discussed the required issues with the patient.

88. C: When using the Z-track method of intramuscular injection, the skin and subcutaneous tissue should be pulled 2.5 to 3.5 cm (1 to 1.4 inches). The Z-track method should be used for all intramuscular injections because it effectively seals the medication into the muscle. A new needle should be placed on the syringe after the syringe is filled. The skin and subcutaneous tissue over the injection site are pulled laterally or downward and held during the injection. The needle should be left in place for 10 seconds after injection to allow the medication to disperse, and then the needle is removed and the skin is released.

89. A: If a patient nearing death has developed noisy gurgling respirations ("death rales"), the nurse's first action should be to slightly elevate the patient's head. These rales develop as secretions pool in the airways and usually indicate that death will occur within 72 hours. Suctioning should be avoided because it is of little help and may increase the patient's discomfort. Anticholinergic medications may be administered to dry the secretions, but they primarily benefit the family or others who find the rales distressing.

90. D: If a patient was recently diagnosed with diabetes mellitus, type 1, and is very stressed about handling the disease, discussing fears and anxiety with the nurse is an example of emotion-focused coping. This important aspect of coping, which can also include activities to take the patient's mind off of the disease, is sometimes overlooked in favor of problem-focused coping strategies, such as attending diabetes education classes, reading about the disease, and working with a nutritionist.

91. C: If a patient is unable to swallow a capsule that contains beaded medication, the nurse should empty the capsule into a small measured volume of syrup or one to two teaspoons of other food (such as gelatin or jelly). The volume should be small to ensure that all is ingested. Beaded medications are enteric-coated and should not be crushed. Because capsules readily dissolve, most capsules can be opened if patients cannot swallow the capsule whole.

92. A: When communicating with an older adult with chronic illness, the nurse should treat the patient as a competent adult. Although short-term memory may be somewhat impaired with age, cognition usually remains stable unless the patient has a disease, such as Alzheimer's, that impairs cognition. Older patients should be encouraged to participate in care planning and treatments and should make their own decisions and do not need to be protected by withholding information.

93. B: In the chain of infection, the source of microorganisms is the reservoir. The six links include

- Etiologic agent: Microorganism causing disease.
- Reservoir: Source of microorganism.
- Portal of exit from reservoir: In humans, this may be the respiratory system, urinary tract, gastrointestinal (GI) tract, blood, tissue, or the reproductive tract.
- Method of transmission: Direct, vehicle-borne, vector-borne, or airborne.
- Portal of entry to host: Break in skin, open tracts.
- Susceptible host: That at risk of infection.

94. D: If a patient frequently climbs out of bed at night to go to the bathroom, the best solution is likely to schedule toileting. For example, the patient might be awakened and taken to the toilet at 12 midnight and again at 4 or 5 a.m. The scheduled toileting should be based on the frequency and times the patient commonly climbs out of bed. If patients climb over the rails, the bed should always be left in the low position and the side rails left in the down position, or alarms (such as the Ambularm) can be used.

95. A: In the immediate postoperative period after extubation, the respiratory rate should be between 10 and 30 per minute. A slow respiratory rate (such as 8 per minute) or a very rapid respiratory rate may both result in impaired oxygenation and should be reported to the physician. Prolonged ventilation during surgery may impair lung function, so the patient should be carefully monitored and chest excursion should be evaluated as well as pulse oximetry performed. Patients usually receive oxygen until their respiratory status has stabilized.

96. D: If a patient tells the nurse, "The doctor has put a camera in my room to watch everything that I do," she is experiencing a delusion of persecution because she may feel threatened in some way. Delusions are personal beliefs that are false and not reality based, and patients often cling to their delusions despite their irrational nature and in the face of obvious proof that the delusions are false. Delusions may occur with psychiatric or neurological disorders.

97. A: The Braden scale is used to predict pressure ulcers. Scoring is based on six categories. The first five categories are scored from 1 to 4 with 1 indicating the most serious impairment and 4 indicating no impairment: sensory perception, moisture, activity, mobility, and nutrition. The last category is friction and shear, and it is scored from 1 to 3 with 1 indicating a problem, 2 a potential problem, and 3 no apparent problem. Total scores can range from 6 to 23 with scores below 19 indicating moderate to severe risk.

98. A, B, and **D:** If a patient has been receiving digoxin (Lanoxin) 0.5 mg per day, but the nurse is concerned that the patient is exhibiting signs of digitoxicity, the indications of digitoxicity include tachycardia or bradycardia and any other type of dysrhythmia. Patients may exhibit central nervous system effects, including confusion, headache, seizures, fatigue, and malaise. Patients may complain of colored vision, halo vision, or flickering lights. Nausea, vomiting, anorexia, and diarrhea are also common.

99. B: Most adults should sleep 7 to 8 hours each night (or at one time if the individual works during the night). Fewer than 6 hours for an adult younger than 65 and fewer than 5 hours for an adult older than age 65 are considered inadequate. The National Sleep Foundation's recommendations include

Age	Recommended	May be ok for some	Not recommended
14 to 17	8 to 10 hours	7 hours, 11 hours	< 7 or >12
18 to 25	7 to 9 hours	6 hours, 11 hours	<6 or >11
26 to 64	7 to 9 hours	6 hours, 10 hours	<6 or >10
≥65	7 to 8 hours	5 to 6 hours, 9 hours	<5 or >9

100. C: When removing an artificial eye, the nurse's first action should be to retract the lower eyelid, using the thumb or first finger of the dominant hand. Then the nurse exerts slight pressure under the eyelid and slides the prosthesis out. If the prosthesis adheres to the socket and does not loosen easily, a moistened suction device can be used to apply some traction to the prosthesis to aid in removal. The nurse should place a towel below the patient's face in case the prosthesis falls during removal.

101. D: If a patient has cirrhosis of the liver and is prescribed medications, metabolism of the medications is most likely to be impaired. Drugs that are primarily broken down for elimination in the liver are most likely to accumulate in the system and can cause overdose or toxic reactions. Medication dosages may need to be modified for those with cirrhosis, or different medications should be selected. Response to drugs may also be altered by cirrhosis. Some drugs such as angiotensin-converting enzyme (ACE) inhibitors and nonsteroidal anti-inflammatory drugs (NSAIDs) should be avoided.

102. A: If the nurse experiences a needlestick injury after giving a patient an injection, his initial response should be to wash the wound with soap and water. As soon as possible, the incident must be reported to a supervisor and steps should be taken according to established protocol. This may include testing and/or prophylaxis, depending on the patient's health history. In some cases, the patient may also be tested for communicable diseases, such as human immunodeficiency virus (HIV), in order to determine the risk to the nurse.

103. D: 1000 grams is equivalent to 1 kilogram.

1/1000	1/100	1/10	Base	× 10	× 100	× 1000
milligram	centigram	decigram	gram	dekagram	hectogram	kilogram

104. A, B, and **C:** Risk factors for sleep apnea include obesity, age over 66, and smoking. Having a sedentary lifestyle (although it may contribute to obesity) by itself is not a risk factor. Those who are obese have a four times higher risk of developing sleep apnea than those of normal weight. Other factors include craniofacial abnormalities that affect airway, acromegaly, and neck circumference greater than 17 inches (because this tends to narrow the airway). Sleep apnea is also more common in males, African-Americans, and those with diabetes and hypertension.

105. B: If a prescription for a wafer calls for "buccal administration," the nurse should place the wafer against the mucous membranes of the cheek so that it can dissolve and be absorbed. The patient should be advised to avoid drinking liquid until the medication is completely dissolved and

to avoid swallowing the medication. Medications that are labels as "sublingual," such as nitroglycerin, are placed under the tongue to dissolve.

106. C: If a patient complains of insomnia but naps for two hours in the afternoon and dozes on and off during the evening, the best solution is probably to stay awake during the daytime. This sleep pattern disrupts the usual sleep-wake cycle to the point that sleeping in the daytime instead of at night becomes the new normal. The patient must work to break this cycle and may need to change activities or set alarms to prevent day sleeping until a new pattern of sleeping at night is established.

107. B: If a patient is receiving heparin therapy, the activated partial thromboplastin time (aPTT) should generally range from 45 to 70 seconds (normal values range from 25 to 35 seconds). The aPTT at therapeutic levels indicates decreased levels of clotting factors and decreased risk of clot formation. If a patient is receiving continuous infusions of heparin, blood can be drawn for testing at any time, but with intermittent administration, the aPTT should be done an hour before the next scheduled dose.

108. D: If a malignant tumor is categorized as stage 3, this generally means that the tumor has spread regionally to adjacent lymph nodes and muscles. Tumors are categorized according to spread in a range from stage 1 (localized) to stage 4 (metastasized to distant organs). Tumors are also categorized according to grade, which is based on the degree of abnormality of the cells (that is how closely they resemble normal cells). For example, if a tumor is stage 1 but grade 3, this means that the tumor is localized, but the cells are poorly differentiated and are likely to spread quickly.

109. 0.125 mg. If levothyroxine is prescribed at 125 micrograms, the equivalent dosage in milligrams is 0.125 mg. Micrograms are converted to milligrams by dividing the micrograms by 1000.

$$125/1000 = 0.125 \text{ mg.}$$

110. C: One tablespoon contains approximately 15 to 16 mL. The tablespoon is a standard American measurement that is used for both wet and dry measurement. One tablespoon of dry measure is approximately equal to one-half ounce or 14.3 g. Although the tablespoon measurement is not commonly used for medications, patients in the home environment often prefer to use teaspoon and tablespoon measures for liquids because they are more familiar with them than with the metric system.

111. A: If a patient believes that insects are crawling all over her skin, the type of hallucination that the patient is experiencing is tactile. Hallucinations are false sensory perceptions and may be auditory, visual, gustatory, or olfactory. Hallucinations can occur with many diseases, including Parkinson's disease (50%), Alzheimer's disease, schizophrenia (70%), epilepsy, and brain tumors. Some medications may cause people to hallucinate, and hallucinations may also occur during withdrawal associated with substance abuse.

112. A and C: When counseling a 26-year-old sexually active HIV-positive male about safe sex practices, the nurse should recommend masturbation and mutual masturbation as well as consistent condom use. Although sexual abstinence is the only sure safe sex practice, suggesting this to a sexually-active 26-year-old patient is probably nonrealistic. The patient should be advised to use a condom with all partners, whether they are HIV positive or not because there are different strains of HIV and viral loads vary.

41

113. D: If a patient indicates on admission for surgery that she will accept no blood products, the patient probably is a Jehovah's Witness. Members are allowed to receive fractionated blood cells, so they may receive hemoglobin-based blood substitutes. The following guidelines are provided to church members:

Basic blood standards for Jehovah's Witnesses	
Not acceptable	Whole blood: red cells, white cells, platelets, plasma
Acceptable	Fractions from red cells, white cells, platelets, and plasma

114. C: When administering a dosage of medication through a metered-dose inhaler (MDI), the dispenser should be held two inches in front of the lips. The MDI should be shaken before each puff. The patient should be instructed to exhale first and then to dispense a dose while inhaling and then to hold the breath for about 10 seconds before exhaling slowing through the lips. The patient should wait one to three minutes between doses, breathing normally. The patient should rinse the mouth with water after completion.

115. A: A spontaneous pneumothorax with accumulation of air in the pleural space occurring with no external wound is categorized as a closed pneumothorax. A closed pneumothorax may occur when small blebs at the surface of the lungs rupture, causing air to leak into the pleural space. Risk increases with heavy smoking (greater than 22 cigarettes daily). A closed pneumothorax may also result from trauma, such as fractured ribs, or from mechanical ventilation.

116. 50 drops per minute. If a patient is to receive 1000 mL of dextrose 5% in water (D5W) over five hours with a drop factor of 15 drops per milliliter, the flow rate should be 50 drops per minute:

- Volume × drop factor/time in minutes = drops per minute.
- $1000 \times 15/300 = 15{,}000/300 = 150/3 = 50$ drops per minute.

117. B: If a patient criticizes another nurse, stating that the nurse refuses to answer any of his questions, the best response is "Let's see if I can help you." It's better to deal with the problem itself—unanswered questions—than to attempt to make excuses, even if what the patient is saying is untrue. When patients are under stress, they may misconstrue the words or actions of healthcare providers, and patients may not always be clear in what they want or need.

118. C: If a patient receives regular insulin (Humulin R, Novalin R, Velosulin BR) on a sliding scale four times a day, it should generally be administered about 30 minutes prior to a scheduled meal. Regular insulin is short acting (30 to 60 minutes) and is the only insulin that can be given intravenously, so regular insulin is used to treat diabetic ketoacidosis. Rapid-acting insulins, such as insulin lispro and insulin aspart, more closely mimic endogenous insulin and are given within 15 minutes of beginning a meal.

119. Two tablets. If a digoxin order is for 0.25 mg, but the medication is provided in 0.125 mg tablets, then the nurse should administer two tablets: $0.25/0.125 = 2$. Although scored pills may be cut in half fairly easily for administration, it is safer to use medications that are the exact dosage in order to decrease the risk of error. Pills that are enteric coated must be administered whole because cutting them may interfere with absorption. In some cases, patients may find it more cost effective to cut pills in half because different dosages may cost about the same.

120. A: Following the death of a patient, the nurse's first step in postmortem care should be to confirm organ donation status because patients who are organ donors may require immediate special procedures. Confirming status also includes determining if the family members have been approached by the organ donation nurse coordinator. Then, the nurse should collect any specimens that might be needed and remove tubes and drains. The nurse should ask the family members if they want to help to prepare the body.

121. B: If a nurse is to administer a medication intramuscularly (IM) to an adult, the site that is preferred is the ventrogluteal, especially if the patient is quite thin. This site is preferred because there are no large nerves or blood vessels that may be inadvertently punctured. Fat content is also lower in this area than in other sites, reducing the chance that the IM medication is administered subcutaneously. The deltoid muscle may be adequate for larger adults.

122. D: If a patient with diabetes mellitus, type 1, complains of increasing thirst and abdominal pain and exhibits tachycardia, orthostatic hypotension, and Kussmaul respirations, the point-of-care testing that should be carried out immediately is blood glucose. These symptoms are consistent with diabetic ketoacidosis, which is blood glucose of greater than 250 mg/dL. Ketonuria is present, but the urine ketone test is less reliable than blood glucose for diagnosis. Immediate treatment includes IV access and fluid and electrolyte replacement, especially potassium because hypokalemia is common, and short-acting insulin.

123. A: An absolute contraindication for a 65-year-old man wanting a prescription for sildenafil (Viagra) for erectile dysfunction is the use of a nitroglycerin transdermal patch (TransDerm-Nitro) or any nitrate product. Nitrates are vasodilators, as is sildenafil; the combination can cause an abrupt drop in blood pressure. Although beta-blockers also have vasodilatory properties, they can usually be taken with sildenafil without a problem. However, the erectile dysfunction may, in fact, be caused by the beta-blocker.

124. B: When a patient is crutch walking, the crutches should be held six inches away from the side of the foot and six inches forward because this provides the best base of support. If the crutches are too close or too far away, the patient is at an increased risk of falling. Typical crutch walking gaits include the two-point gait, the three-point gait, the four-point gait, and the swing-through gait. The gait is selected depending on the type of injury and the patient's body strength.

125. A: If a patient has a chest tube in place and experiences a sudden decrease in drainage, the nurse's first action should be to check the drainage system for obstruction/kinking because this is the most common reason for a sudden change. In some cases, clots may be blocking the tube. If the tube appears patent and no blockage is found that can be remedied, a thorough respiratory assessment should be carried out, observing for a mediastinal shift or respiratory distress (both indicating a medical emergency), and the change should be reported to the physician.

126. D: When assisting a patient with a bed bath, the area of the body that should be washed last is the perineum. The general rule is that the patient is bathed from "clean to dirty," and the perineal area could be contaminated with fecal material. The bath usually begins with the face and progresses to the arms and hands, chest and abdomen, legs and feet, back, and then the perineum. Bed bathwater should be maintained between 110° and 115° F.

127. B: Paralysis associated with Guillain-Barré syndrome is usually ascending. Weakness usually begins in the lower extremities over a variable period of time (hours to weeks) with symptoms usually peaking at about 14 days. Patients may experience numbness and tingling as well as hypotonia and areflexia. The paralysis may affect the muscles of respiration, leading to respiratory failure, so some patients must be intubated and maintained on mechanical ventilation. Treatment includes supportive care and plasmapheresis or high-dose immunoglobulin.

128. C: Patients should avoid using nasal spray decongestants, such as oxymetazoline (Afrin), for more than 10 days because of the risk of rebound congestion. Antihistamines may relieve nasal congestion associated with allergies. Patients with long-term or chronic nasal congestion may have better results from nasal corticosteroids, such as Nasacort or Flonase. Other conservative treatments include using a humidifier, taking a hot shower, and using a neti pot.

129. C: If a patient is receiving oxygen therapy per nasal cannula, the maximum flow rate is 6 L/min. Above that, there is no improvement in inspired oxygen concentration (FiO_2), and the increased airflow may dry the mucous membranes. Humidification must be used with flow rates of 4 L/min and higher. The nasal cannula is simple to use and more comfortable for most patients than other delivery systems; however, if the patient is a mouth breather, this can affect the FiO_2, and the nasal cannula is contraindicated with nasal obstruction.

130. A: Leukotriene receptor antagonists, such as montelukast (Singulair), are used for prophylaxis and long-term treatment of asthma. Leukotrienes are produced by the body in response to an allergic response. In patients with asthma, these leukotrienes cause inflammation, bronchoconstriction, and increased mucus production, leading to the classic symptoms of asthma: wheezing, coughing, and dyspnea. Leukotriene receptor antagonists prevent the leukotrienes from attaching to receptors in the immune system, thus reducing inflammation and asthma symptoms.

131. C: If a patient is to have ice packs applied intermittently to an ankle four times daily, the maximum duration each time should be 20 to 30 minutes. If circulation is impaired, then the duration should be less. The ice pack should not come directly in contact with the skin because that may cause skin burns. If using ice cubes, enough water should be placed in the pack to just cover the ice because this equalizes the cold throughout the pack and helps the pack mold to the body part.

132. B: The oxygen delivery system that best controls the specific oxygen concentration (up to 60%) is the Venturi mask. The air is humidified, so this system does not dry the mucous membranes. However, the Venturi mask must be properly fitted and it can be hot and confining for many patients. Patients have difficulty communicating with the Venturi mask and are unable to eat while receiving oxygen therapy because the mask covers the nose, mouth, and chin.

133. A: According to Freud's psychosocial development theory, the agency of the mind that is responsible for all drives and operates on the pleasure principle is the id, which is present at birth and operates in response to discomfort and hunger. The id seeks to reduce tension. The ego is evident during the fourth or fifth month of life and helps the infant distinguish the external world from the internal. The ego operates on the reality principle and facilitates reality testing. The superego develops between ages three and five from interactions with others. The conscience is part of the superego.

134. B: A normal BMI ranges from 18.5 to 24.9 kg/m³. BMI for adults

Weight classification	BMI range
Underweight	<18.5 kg/m³
Normal weight	18.5 to 24.9 kg/m³
Overweight	25 to 29.9 kg/m³
Obese, class I (severe)	30 to 34.9 kg/m³
Obese, class II (morbid)	35 to 39.9 kg/m³
Obese, class III (extreme)	≥ 40 kg/m³

135. A and C: In middle adulthood (about ages 40 to 60), individuals tend to achieve career satisfaction but may begin to reassess priorities of life. Social involvement tends to expand as the individual takes more interest in the world in general with less focus on the self. Individuals may assist children and others in the next generation to gain maturity. This is also a period of beginning decline in physical skills, muscle strength, and stamina. Chronic health problems, such as hypertension and diabetes, are common.

136. C: The most common cause of COPD is a history of smoking because smoking causes severe damage to pulmonary tissues. Smoking causes emphysema because it damages the walls of the alveoli so that it's more difficult to absorb oxygen or rid the body of carbon dioxide. Smoking also causes chronic inflammation of the airways with thickening of the walls and increased mucus production, resulting in chronic bronchitis. Both of these conditions are present with COPD. If patients continue to smoke with COPD, the smoking may result in exacerbations.

137. D: If a 17-year-old burn patient who is normally even-tempered becomes frustrated while undergoing a painful dressing change and throws a screaming tantrum, the defense mechanism that the patient is exhibiting is regression. The patient has retreated to an earlier stage of development because this provides some measure of relief from the discomfort the patient is experiencing. The nurse should acknowledge the patient's frustration without making judgmental statements about the patient's behavior: "I can see this is really stressful for you."

138. B: When irrigating or cleansing a wound, the most commonly used solution is normal saline. Normal saline is not associated with adverse effects and does not affect healing. If the wound is grossly contaminated, then betadine solution is sometimes used, but this should be thoroughly rinsed from the wound with normal saline. Hydrogen peroxide (3%) is also sometimes used to remove debris from a wound, but it may impede healing and should be followed by a normal saline rinse.

139. C: According to Kübler-Ross, the stage of grief that a patient is likely undergoing if the patient, who has been diagnosed with cancer, begins to pray daily and to attend church regularly is bargaining. Essentially, the patient is bargaining with God to reverse or delay loss. The patient may feel guilty for past actions and feel that the cancer is a punishment from God. The patient may feel a temporary sense of hope during the bargaining stage, and this period may give the patient time to accept the reality of the diagnosis.

140. A and C: If a patient is on dysphagia pureed diet (level 1), orange juice with pulp and pureed strawberries should be avoided. Foods that are allowed include drinks (without pulp and thickened to the prescribed consistency if necessary); pureed meats, eggs, and legumes; hot cereals and pureed pastries and bread products; applesauce and pureed fruit without skin or seeds; pureed vegetables (without seed or skin); mashed potatoes; refried beans, strained soups (thickened as necessary); and desserts such as gelatin, custard, yogurt, and pudding.

141. B: If a patient who is newly diagnosed with Parkinson's disease is overcome with anxiety and despair, constantly worrying about his ability to cope when his condition deteriorates in the future, he is experiencing anticipatory grief. The patient is expressing profound grief before the loss actually occurs. Some degree of anticipatory grief is normal in response to future loss and may actually shorten the later grieving process, but if the process occurs too early or is prolonged, it can interfere with the patient's ability to cope and can hasten loss.

142. A: Organic material, such as blood and fecal material, should be cleansed from objects and surfaces prior to application of a disinfectant primary to prevent inactivation of the disinfectant. This can occur with disinfectants such as alcohol. Cleansing also helps to prevent residue buildup.

The manufacturer's directions should be followed regarding the concentration of the disinfectant and the contact time necessary for disinfection.

143. C: If the nurse plans to use a bladder scanner to assess a patient's residual urinary retention, the scan should be done within 10 to 15 minutes of urination. The bladder scanner must be set for male or female patients, but if a female patient has had a hysterectomy, the male setting should be used. About 30 mL of conductivity gel should be applied about 3 cm above the symphysis pubis and the scan head placed directly on the gel, making sure that the directional icon points toward the patient's head. The probe should be applied with steady, light pressure and should be pointed downward.

144. D: When changing a patient's colostomy bag following surgery, if the nurse notes that the stoma appears dark purple, the nurse should notify the physician because this color is not normal. The stoma should be pink or red, but if it changes color to blue, purple, or gray-tinged, this can indicate impaired circulation to the stoma and cyanosis, and these can lead to necrosis. Ischemia is most commonly noted within the first 24 postoperative hours. If not severe, it may be treated conservatively, but in some cases the patient may need to return for surgical repair.

145. 7.5 mL. If a patient is to receive 3 mg of albuterol sulfate syrup four times daily, and the syrup contains 2 mg per 5 mL, then the patient should receive 7.5 mL for each dose. Formula:

- Milligrams needed/milligrams available × volume
- $3/2 = 1.5 \times 5 = 7.5$ mL.

146. B: If a patient engages in running, which is a vigorous aerobic exercise, for 75 minutes per week, the patient should engage in strength training twice weekly. No specific recommendation is made regarding the time spent doing strength training. Those who engage in moderate aerobic exercise, such as brisk walking or swimming, should exercise for 150 minutes per week. Patients should, however, be encouraged to exercise 30 minutes daily. This period of exercise may be done at one time or broken up into shorter periods of exercise.

147. D: The nurse should avoid lifting heavy items that weigh more than 50 lb. Even this weight may be excessive for some people, especially those with back injuries or osteoporosis. When lifting, the nurse should be careful to avoid leaning forward or reaching up to lift because this puts extra strain on the muscles. Items that are too heavy should not be lifted manually, but they should be lifted with a lifting device or with the assistance of another person.

148. C: If a patient has frostbite on both hands, the most likely treatment is immersing the hands in warm water, ranging in temperature from 37° C to 40° C (98.6° F to 104° F). Circulating water with controlled temperature is most effective. The baths are done for 30 to 40 minutes at a time and then repeated until circulation is restored. Massage or excessive handling may damage the tissue. Once the part is rewarmed, it may swell, so it must be elevated and protected from pressure.

149. A: When cleansing instruments that are contaminated with blood, the instruments should first be rinsed in cold water to remove organic material because it may set if in contact with warm or hot water. After rinsing, the instruments should then be thoroughly washed with soap and water and rinsed being disinfected or sterilized. The nurse should always use contact precautions and wear gloves and gown when handling blood-contaminated instruments.

150. A and B: Signs of immune thrombocytopenic purpura (ITP) include petechia, ecchymosis, and epistaxis. ITP is an autoimmune disorder in which platelets are destroyed at an abnormal rate because the body's immune system attacks the cells. Production of platelets may also be impaired.

Because platelets are essential for clotting, this results in increased risk for bleeding. Patients are often asymptomatic, although hemorrhage can occur if levels fall below 20,000 (the normal range is 150,000 to 450,000).

151. B: If a patient experiences frequent ingrown toenails, the nurse can suspect that the patient uses incorrect nail trimming technique. Whereas fingernails are trimmed to the shape of the finger, toenails should be trimmed straight across. Ingrown toenails may also be an indication of tight, poorly fitting shoes. Women who wear very high heels with pointed toes risk developing ingrown toenails. Patients with ingrown toenails should be referred to a podiatrist, especially those who are diabetic or have impaired peripheral circulation.

152. C: About 66% of the body water is located in the intracellular space, which is within the cells. This is classified as intracellular fluid (ICF) and constitutes about 40% of the total body weight. The rest of the body water is classified as extracellular fluid (ECF) and comprises interstitial fluid (fluid in the space between cells) and transcellular fluid (fluid in specialized cavities such as peritoneal fluid). ECF is found in the intravascular space as well as the interstitium and transcellular spaces.

153. A: The electrolytes that are most prevalent in the extracellular fluid (ECF) are sodium (which is an anion carrying a negative charge) and chloride (which is a cation carrying a positive charge). The ECF also contains small amounts of the cations potassium, magnesium, and calcium and the anions bicarbonate, sulfate, and phosphate. Cations and anions combine to ensure that there is a balance between negative and positive ions. In intracellular fluid (ICF), on the other hand, potassium (cation) and phosphate (anion) are most prevalent.

154. B: Frequent contact with latex may increase the risk of developing an allergic response. People who are especially at risk are healthcare workers and patients who have had frequent hospitalizations, prolonged use of equipment or materials containing latex (such as catheters), or frequent surgical procedures. People who work in industries in which they come in contact with latex or natural rubber are also at risk.

155. D: Cobalamin (vitamin B_{12}) is not absorbed with pernicious anemia. Normally, gastric mucosa secretes intrinsic factor, which is required for absorption of cobalamin. With pernicious anemia, antibodies have attacked the cells producing the intrinsic factor or attacked the intrinsic factor itself. Onset is usually after age 40 (most commonly at age 60), and it occurs primarily in people of northern European or African-American heritage. Symptoms include red, sore, beefy tongue; nausea; vomiting; abdominal pain; weakness; paresthesia; and ataxia. Cobalamin is administered parenterally or intranasally, usually once a month after the condition has stabilized.

156. C: If a patient with COPD has been eating poorly because eating exhausts her, she should be advised to rest for 30 minutes before meals. Additionally, the patient should be encouraged to eat frequent small meals rather than three large meals. Patients with COPD often have increased cough in the morning because of the pooling of secretions during sleep, so most patients should have their largest meal at a later time, such as midday.

157. B: The movement of molecules from an area of high concentration to one of low concentration is referred to as diffusion. Diffusion can occur in liquids, gases, and solids. If a membrane separates molecules, then the membrane must be permeable in order for diffusion to occur. Movement across the membrane stops when the concentration on both sides equalizes. In some cases, special carrier molecules increase the rate of diffusion, resulting in facilitated (or faster) diffusion, which occurs with glucose.

158. A: When speaking with the spouse of a patient from Latin America, if the nurse feels uncomfortable because the spouse stands very close when talking to him, the person is exhibiting a cultural pattern. Proxemics (the way people use space) vary among cultures. While most Americans feel comfortable keeping an arm's length separating them from others when conversing, some cultures (notably Middle Eastern and Latin American) prefer to stand closer. Others, such as Asian cultures, prefer an even greater distance.

159. C: If an electrical fire erupts on the unit, the fire extinguisher that is used must be labeled for type C fires. Types of fires include

- Class A: Ordinary fires involving such things as wood, paper, and trash.
- Class B: Fires involving flammable liquids.
- Class C: Electrical fires.
- Class D: Fires of combustible metals, such as potassium or lithium.
- Class K: Cooking oil, vegetable oil, or animal fat fires.

160. A: If a Chinese patient insists on keeping very warm despite the heat and avoids certain foods that she describes as "cold" even though they are, in fact, warm, the patient is probably trying to keep yin and yang in balance, that is, hot and cold elements. Chinese and Vietnamese cultures believe that when yin and yang are out of balance, illness results. Being hot or cold does not necessarily correlate with actual temperature because some cold foods may be classified as hot and some hot as cold.

161. A: With gonorrhea, the infected female is usually asymptomatic in the initial stages but develops symptoms later when the disease progresses to infection of the cervix, urethra, and fallopian tubes. Men, on the other hand, often exhibit acute symptoms that include urethritis with purulent discharge, dysuria, proctitis, and pharyngitis. In females, gonorrhea may result in chronic pelvic inflammatory disease, infertility, and ectopic pregnancy, whereas males may become sterile. Gonorrhea is spread through vaginal, anal, and oral sex. Eyes may become infected from contaminated hands.

162. D: If a patient is diagnosed with body lice, he should be advised to wash all clothes and linens in hot water (130° F) and to dry them in a hot dryer. Body lice are spread through direct physical contact or contact with clothing or other articles (linens, towels) that have been in contact with an infested patient. Treatment is with a pediculicide (such as Kwell). Patients should be aware that lice can spread through contact with upholstered furniture and fabric toys as well. The home should be thoroughly vacuumed and cleaned.

163. C: If a patient is being treated for anorexia, a reasonable goal for weight gain each week is two to three pounds until the patient has reached at least 80% of the normal body weight for the person's age and size. The patient must be carefully observed to ensure that she is not using laxatives or vomiting to reduce intake and absorption and that she is not stashing food to discard later. In order to be successful, treatment must include psychological therapy to help the patient develop a more realistic self-image.

164. A and B: According to Maslow, self-actualized individuals have an appropriate perception of reality and are able to concentrate on solving problems. They also have the ability to respond spontaneously and do not always conform to expectations. Self-actualized individuals are accepting of themselves and others and identify with humankind. They tend to be independent and to act with autonomy. Self-actualization is the pinnacle of Maslow's hierarchy of needs, but many people never reach this stage.

165. A: With sickle cell anemia, sickling episodes are most commonly caused by infection, which results in hypoxia or deoxygenation of red blood cells. Sickling can also be triggered by many other things, including high altitude, physical stress, emotional stress, dehydration, trauma, surgery, or blood loss. Sickled red blood cells take on a rigid sickle shape, making it difficult for them to pass through small capillaries, so they tend to gather in clumps, resulting in a vaso-occlusive crisis, which impairs blood flow and results in severe pain and tissue ischemia.

166. A and **C:** Common sensory effects of aging related to vision include a general decline in vision. The eye lens begins to harden and then impairs accommodation so that people become increasingly farsighted, especially after age 45. The eye lens also tends to yellow, and this interferes with the perception of color. Night vision tends to be somewhat impaired, and the eyes may be more sensitive to glare, such as from oncoming headlights. Cataracts, spots, and floaters are common and may interfere with vision.

167. B: White bread (1 slice) is very low in fiber at 0.6 g because the flour in it is refined. Oatmeal (1/2 cup) and popcorn (3 cups) both contain 2 g. Dried peas and beans are especially high in fiber with black beans (1/2 cup), containing 6.1 g. Light red kidney beans contain 7.9 g. Fruits (1 medium or 1/2 cup berries) average from 2 to 4 g, and vegetables vary from a low of 1.5 for broccoli to 4.5 for brussels sprouts.

168. C: If a patient is taking warfarin (Coumadin), he should avoid consuming green, leafy vegetables in excess because of their vitamin K content. The patient should maintain a stable intake of these vegetables so that the effect on the anticoagulant does not vary. Vitamin K is necessary for synthesis of prothrombin, a critical element in blood clotting; in fact, vitamin K is used as an antidote for excessive anticoagulation. Warfarin interferes with synthesis of vitamin K clotting factors in the liver.

169. D: Smoking cessation is an example of primary prevention because it is carried out in order to prevent the onset of disease rather than to identify or treat the disease. Primary preventive efforts are often aimed at large segments of the population, such as federal guidelines for exercise and diet. However, primary prevention may be aimed at smaller populations as well, such as when a high school offers condoms and counseling about pregnancy prevention to students.

170. B: With polycythemia vera, all types of blood cells are affected: platelets, red blood cells, and white blood cells. Polycythemia vera is a myeloproliferative disorder that results from a chromosomal abnormality, the reason that it affects all cells instead of just red blood cells. Hypervolemia and hyperviscosity occur and can lead to various symptoms, including headache, itching (from increased basophils), tinnitus, visual disturbances, paresthesias, and burning and redness of hands and feet. The primary treatment is phlebotomy.

171. A: If a patient with arthritis complains of bilateral tinnitus, aspirin may be the cause. It is unclear why aspirin causes tinnitus, but usually a high dosage (eight or more tablets daily) is required to cause this effect, which is generally reversible when the medication is discontinued or dose lowered, so low-dose aspirin is not usually a risk factor. Tinnitus is an often constant ringing or buzzing sound in the ears. Others nonsteroidal anti-inflammatory drugs (NSAIDs), such as ibuprofen, have also been linked to tinnitus.

172. C: The term for personal standards regarding what is right or wrong is *morality*. Issues of morality generally are those that involve social values and societal norms rather than common everyday matters. The term *ethics* is often used interchangeably with *morality*, but *ethics* refers to the method of inquiry about what is right or wrong or the beliefs of a group as a whole rather than the individual. Bioethics refers specifically to ethical issues regarding life.

173. D: The moral principle (which is a broad general concept) that decrees that the nurse should do no harm when providing care to a patient is nonmaleficence. However, in some cases, treatments may have a harmful effect. For example, a dressing change to improve healing may result in pain. In this case, beneficence (carrying out an action to benefit the patient) is in conflict with nonmaleficence. A moral dilemma can occur when two moral principles are in conflict with each other.

174. B, C, and **D:** For fall prevention, tripping hazards such as throw rugs, loose carpets, and other obstacles should be removed. Lighting should be bright, especially around stairways. Grab bars should be installed in the bathrooms and other key areas. The home should be checked to ensure that no electrical cords run across walkways. Beds should be at the right height, and chairs should be stable. It is probably not realistic to recommend that a patient move to a home that is all on one level, and the lack of stairs does not by itself make for a safe environment.

175. B: If the nurse is bathing a patient and the patient repeatedly tells the nurse to stop touching her, failing to do so could be considered battery. Battery involves intentionally touching an individual or the individual's clothing or items the individual is holding after the individual tells the person to stop. This touching must be wrong or cause harm in some way, such as when done without permission or when causing injury, shame, or embarrassment.

176. D: Nursing practice is governed by the state nurse practice act. Each state and territory has its own nurse practice act that governs nursing practice. Although these acts tend to be similar, there are some variations. Nurse practice acts may be influenced by professional nursing organizations, and the place of employment may put limitations on practice that exceed those of the nurse practice act. For example, a hospital may not allow a practical nurse to administer medications even though this is within their scope of practice according to the nurse practice act of the state.

177. If a patient weighs 136.4 pounds, this is equivalent to 62 kilograms. There are 2.2 pounds in each kilogram, so 136.4/2.2 = 62. Although most people in the United States calculate their weight according to the United States standard, which uses pounds and ounces, the metric system is used almost exclusively for medical purposes.

178. C: If a nurse is assigned to care for a patient and drops the Foley catheter on an unsterile surface before inserting it, resulting in a urinary tract infection and sepsis, the action would be classified as malpractice because it meets the four necessary conditions:

- The nurse was assigned to provide care to the patient.
- The nurse violated a standard of care (using a contaminated catheter).
- The patient experienced harm (urinary infection and sepsis).
- The harm was caused directly by the nurse's failure to observe a standard to which the nurse was aware.

179. B: A common finding with left-sided heart failure is paroxysmal nocturnal dyspnea. With left-sided heart failure, the left side of the heart does not function adequately, so blood backs up in the lungs. Because of this, many of the symptoms relate to pulmonary function and include dyspnea, orthopnea, and signs of inadequate oxygenation. Rales may be heard at the bases of the lungs. Cerebral hypoxia or anoxia may result in confusion and disorientation.

180. D: If a nurse threatens a patient with restraints if the patient doesn't stop complaining, this could be considered an assault, which can be an actual act that involves touching a patient against his or her will or the threat to do so. If the nurse followed through and applied the restraints, this could be considered an act of false imprisonment. It's important to remember that patients do not lose rights simply because they are ill or disruptive.

181. C: If a patient has a left trochanteric pressure ulcer that is full thickness with exposed subcutaneous tissue and slough, the pressure ulcer would be classified as stage III. Stages:

- Suspected: Blood blister, discolored skin, pain, texture change, or temperature change.
- Stage I: Localized, nonblanching reddened area.
- Stage II: Partial thickness skin loss involving epidermis and dermis. Abrasion/Blistered appearance.
- Stage III: As above. Without exposure of muscle or bone.
- Stage IV: Extends to muscle, bone, tendons, or joints with extensive damage and necrosis.
- Unstageable: Slough and/or eschar in wound makes staging impossible until debridement.

182. B: When applying warm compresses, the nurse recognizes that maximal vasodilation occurs within 20 to 30 minutes, so treatments are usually limited to this duration but are repeated intermittently. Moist heat compresses penetrate deep muscles better than dry heat, such as from a heating pad. The temperature of warm compresses should be checked before application. Patients with diabetes, stroke, spinal cord injury, rheumatoid arthritis, and neuropathy may have reduced sensation and are especially at risk for burns.

183. 66 beats per minute. If a patient's heart rate recorded over a week from Sunday to Saturday was 66, 62, 72, 70, 74, 64, and 60, the patient's median heart rate was 66. To find the median rate, the first step is to put the numbers in order from lowest to highest:

60, 62, 64, 66, 70, 72, 74

The middle number (the number that has an equal number below it and above it) is the median, in this case 66 because three numbers are lower and three numbers are higher.

184. A: If the goal for a patient is "Patient will have relief from pain," an appropriate desired outcome is "Patient will express fewer verbal/nonverbal indications of pain" because this is in some way measurable either directly through counting interactions or through observation. "Patient will be free of pain" and "Patient will appear comfortable" are subjective, whereas "Patient will ask for pain medication less often" does not necessarily mean that the patient has relief from pain.

Practice Test #2

1. If a patient with a history of asthma is experiencing an acute exacerbation with wheezing and dyspnea, the medication likely to provide the most immediate relief is

    a. prednisone (corticosteroid)

    b. montelukast (leukotriene receptor antagonist).

    c. ipratropium (anticholinergic).

    d. albuterol (beta-adrenergic agonist).

2. Patients with gynoid (pear-shaped) obesity have increased risk of

    a. breast cancer.

    b. varicose veins.

    c. heart disease.

    d. diabetes mellitus.

3. Which of the following increases the risk of pulmonary embolus in the postoperative period?

    a. Hypocoagulability.

    b. Age younger than 60.

    c. Prolonged immobilization.

    d. Thyroid disease.

4. A patient who has undergone a colectomy for a bowel obstruction is refusing to turn, get out of bed, or cooperate. Which assessment has priority?

    a. Pain.

    b. Wound.

    c. Vital signs.

    d. Emotional status.

5. A patient has diabetic ketoacidosis, and her arterial blood gases are

- pH 7.22.
- $PaCO_2$ 41 mm Hg.
- HCO_3 15 mEq/L.

Which one of the following acid-base imbalances do these findings indicate?

    a. Respiratory acidosis.

    b. Respiratory alkalosis.

    c. Metabolic acidosis.

    d. Metabolic alkalosis.

6. If an Orthodox Jewish patient who is refusing to use electrical appliances on the Sabbath will not use the call bell or respond to the intercom, the nurse should

    a. tell him that exceptions are made for ill patients.

    b. provide him with a hand bell or alternate means of calling the nurse.

    c. check on him every 15 to 30 minutes.

    d. advise him that he is putting himself at risk.

7. In the communication process, *channel* refers to

    a. the means of sending and receiving a message.
    b. the message returned by a receiver.
    c. the factors that influence communication.
    d. the setting in which communication occurs.

8. If a patient with kidney disease is limited to 0.6 mg of protein per kg of body weight and she weighs 165 pounds, how many milligrams of protein is the patient allowed each day?

    _____ mg.

9. Prolonged antibiotic or corticosteroid use increases the risk of

    a. gingivitis.
    b. constipation.
    c. candidiasis.
    d. anaphylaxis.

10. The correct position to place a patient in when he is going into shock is

    a. semi-Fowler's.
    b. reverse Trendelenburg.
    c. flat, supine.
    d. Trendelenburg.

11. The ability of the nurse to listen to a patient, perceive the patient's feelings, and understand the patient's perspectives is an example of

    a. sympathy.
    b. empathy.
    c. patience.
    d. compassion.

12. Which one of the following laboratory test values should the nurse report to the physician because it's outside of the normal range?

    a. Hemoglobin 9.1 g/dL.
    b. Platelets 165,000/mm3.
    c. Hgb A1c 5.5
    d. Glucose 98 g/dL.

13. If the nurse administers a medication to the wrong patient, her priority response should be to

    a. file an incident report.
    b. notify the physician.
    c. assess the patient for an adverse reaction.
    d. notify the supervisor.

14. A patient has had severe watery diarrhea and vomiting for 48 hours. Which electrolyte imbalance is likely to occur with persistent vomiting and diarrhea?

    a. Hypernatremia.
    b. Hyponatremia.
    c. Hypercalcemia.
    d. Hypocalcemia.

15. If a patient is declared brain dead after a motorcycle accident, who should discuss organ donation with the family?

 a. The patient's physician.
 b. Any nurse on duty.
 c. Registered nurses only.
 d. Specially trained personnel.

16. When carrying out range-of-motion exercises, what motions should the patient's elbows go through? **Select all that apply.**

 a. Internal rotation.
 b. Lateral flexion.
 c. Flexion.
 d. Extension.

17. According to Erikson, the primary task of young adults is

 a. autonomy versus shame.
 b. identify versus role confusion.
 c. intimacy versus isolation.
 d. integrity versus despair.

18. Watery wound drainage that is yellow tinged and has occasional red streaks would be categorized as

 a. purulent.
 b. sanguineous.
 c. serous.
 d. serosanguineous.

19. A patient who has been awaiting chemotherapy treatment becomes suddenly very anxious and exhibits rapid pulse, trembling, and diaphoresis. Which response is the most helpful?

 a. "Take deep breaths and relax."
 b. "What were you thinking about right before you started feeling bad?"
 c. "Don't worry. Everything will be fine."
 d. "Try to think of something positive instead of worrying."

20. Which of the following religions forbid the eating of pork? Select all that apply.

 a. Judaism.
 b. Islam.
 c. Latter Day Saints (Mormon).
 d. Hinduism.

21. If a patient is very upset because she is nearing her 65th birthday, the type of crisis the patient is likely experiencing is

 a. life transitional.
 b. traumatic.
 c. maturational.
 d. situational.

22. A patient who has had a stroke with right-sided paralysis has persistent drooling and impaired swallowing. Which type of suctioning is indicated?

   a. Tracheal.
   b. Endotracheal.
   c. Oropharyngeal.
   d. Nasopharyngeal.

23. If a patient is allowed no weight bearing on the left leg, the most appropriate crutch gait is

   a. two-point.
   b. three-point.
   c. four-point.
   d. swing-through.

24. If a patient develops signs of bacterial food poisoning within 30 minutes of eating, the most likely causative agent is

   a. *Clostridium perfringens.*
   b. *Salmonella typhimurium.*
   c. *Clostridium botulinum.*
   d. *Staphylococcus aureus.*

25. Adults should receive the tetanus, diphtheria, and pertussis (Tdap) vaccination

   a. every 10 years.
   b. one time.
   c. annually.
   d. every 5 years.

26. Which cultural/ethnic group is likely to experience a condition referred to as "ghost sickness," which may involve having bad dreams or exhibiting abnormal behavior?

   a. Navajo.
   b. Chinese.
   c. Hispanic.
   d. Hmong.

27. In order to prevent food poisoning, ground beef should be cooked to

   a. 125° F.
   b. 140° F.
   c. 160° F.
   d. 180° F.

28. A patient has nonblanching erythema of intact skin over the coccygeal area. Which of the following treatments may be indicated? Select all that apply.

   a. Frequent turning.
   b. Massage of the reddened area.
   c. Application of alcohol to the reddened area.
   d. Application of transparent dressing over the reddened area.

29. Peak flow meters are used to measure the

   a. airflow after normal exhalation.
   b. airflow after normal inhalation.
   c. highest airflow during forced inhalation.
   d. highest airflow during forced exhalation.

30. A patient has slipped down in the bed and is in an uncomfortable position. Which of the following nursing actions should be avoided?

   a. Use a slip sheet and an assistant to move the patient.
   b. Sit the patient on the side of the bed and have the patient move up.
   c. Grasp the patient under the arms from the head of the bed and pull.
   d. Instruct the patient on the use of the trapeze to change position.

31. Which of the following complications is most common with Crohn's disease?

   a. Rectal bleeding.
   b. Fistulas.
   c. Tenesmus.
   d. Toxic megacolon.

32. Which of the following complementary therapies uses meters and monitors to help patients learn to control bodily functions?

   a. Homeopathy.
   b. Ayurveda.
   c. Acupuncture.
   d. Biofeedback.

33. If a patient complains that something in the abdominal surgical site "gave way" when coughing, and the dressings are immediately saturated with serosanguineous drainage, then the nurse should suspect

   a. dehiscence.
   b. evisceration.
   c. hemorrhage.
   d. normal response to cough.

34. If the nurse is assigned by the supervisor to do a task for which he does not feel prepared, then he should

   a. ask other staff members to help.
   b. attempt to research the task.
   c. tell the supervisor immediately.
   d. refuse to do the task.

35. If a confused patient insists that someone is being tortured when she hears the ambulance siren, the best response is

   a. "No one is being tortured here."
   b. "That noise is an ambulance siren."
   c. "Don't worry; I'll take care of it."
   d. "No one is going to hurt you. You are safe."

36. If a patient weighs 143 pounds and must receive a medication at the rate of 3 mg/kg, how many mg should the patient receive?

_____ mg.

37. If a patient has an ascending colostomy, the consistency of the stool is usually

    a. solid, firm.
    b. semiliquid to soft.
    c. soft formed.
    d. liquid.

38. For nasopharyngeal suctioning of adults, the catheter should be inserted approximately how far?

    a. 6 cm.
    b. 10 cm.
    c. 16 cm.
    d. 20 cm.

39. If a patient has severe ascites, a paracentesis is usually

    a. done only to relieve severe dyspnea or pain.
    b. done routinely every week or so.
    c. avoided under all circumstances.
    d. done as an elective procedure at the patient's request.

40. If a patient is able to respond but does not recall his son's name or the date and doesn't know where he is, the patient could be described as

    a. confused.
    b. disoriented.
    c. psychotic.
    d. delirious.

41. If the nurse is caring for a patient who is receiving a transfusion of platelets because of severe thrombocytopenia, which of the following observations should be reported immediately?

    a. Bruising at the IV puncture site.
    b. Sleepiness and lethargy.
    c. Slight bloody discharge when blowing nose.
    d. Chills and itching.

42. Which of the following are examples of objective data? Select all that apply.

    a. "BP 128/86, pulse 84."
    b. "Erythema extends 2 cm around the wound perimeter."
    c. "Patient complains of headache and dizziness."
    d. "Patient's pain decreased from 8 to 2 on a 1 to 10 scale."

43. Which of the following types of pressure-reducing beds/mattresses may result in increased perspiration and dehydration?

    a. Egg-crate mattress.
    b. Air-suspension bed.
    c. Air-fluidized bed.
    d. Memory foam mattress.

44. If a patient that the nurse is caring for has had continuous IV therapy for four days and the nurse notes that the IV insertion site in his arm is swollen and the tissue is red and tender with a red streak extending proximally, the most likely reason is

a. infiltration.
b. phlebitis.
c. allergic reaction.
d. thrombosis.

45. If a patient has developed a postoperative infection and has a large open wound that must be packed with alginate, the alginate should be

a. packed to above skin level.
b. packed in a single layer only.
c. packed tightly.
d. packed loosely.

46. A patient who is being discharged states she is happy about going home but appears anxious, is wringing her hands, and is avoiding eye contact. Which response is most therapeutic?

a. "I'm sure you'll do fine at home."
b. "I get the feeling that you aren't telling me the truth."
c. "You say you're happy, but you seem anxious."
d. "Are you sure you're ok?"

47. When assisting a patient with overactive bladder to extend time between urinations, if the patient usually urinates every hour, the first goal should be to extend this time by

a. 5 minutes.
b. 15 minutes.
c. 30 minutes.
d. 60 minutes.

48. Bariatric beds are intended for

a. patients who are more than 100 lb. (45 kg) overweight.
b. patients who are malnourished and cachectic.
c. patients in need of pressure reduction.
d. patients taller than 6 feet 5 inches (1.8 m).

49. If a woman tells the nurse that her child has swallowed a poison, the first question should be

a. "How much poison did the child swallow?"
b. "When did the child swallow the poison?"
c. "Did the child vomit after swallowing the poison?"
d. "What poison did the child swallow?"

50. If a patient is developing pneumonia, which stage of the disease is likely to occur first?

a. Resolution.
b. Dilation of capillaries (red hepatization).
c. Congestion.
d. Consolidation (gray hepatization).

51. In the orientation phase of a therapeutic relationship, the primary role of the nurse is to
    a. guide the patient.
    b. build trust.
    c. establish rules of interaction.
    d. take action.

52. Which of the following wound care products is designed to hydrate a wound?
    a. Hydrogel.
    b. Hydrocolloid.
    c. Alginate.
    d. Transparent film.

53. Which of the following is the primary problem with narrative documentation?
    a. It is difficult to do.
    b. It is completed too quickly.
    c. It is impersonal.
    d. It is difficult to retrieve data from.

54. When using the PLISSIT assessment of sexuality, the nurse should always begin the assessment by
    a. asking the patient directly about sexual matters.
    b. waiting for the patient to bring up the topic of sexuality.
    c. asking permission to discuss sexual matters.
    d. telling the patient that some people are uncomfortable discussing sexuality.

55. If a patient is to receive 600 mg of cephalexin oral suspension per nasogastric (NG) tube every six hours, and the oral suspension contains 250mg per 5 mL, how many mL should the nurse administer for each dose?

    _____ mL.

56. Patients with cirrhosis of the liver should be advised that they must maintain abstinence of
    a. caffeinated products.
    b. alcohol.
    c. tobacco products.
    d. fatty foods.

57. An aide reports to the nurse that a patient with pancreatic cancer is complaining of severe abdominal pain and lying rigidly in bed, but the nurse notes that the patient only has an NSAID ordered for pain. The nurse's first action should be to
    a. administer the NSAID.
    b. request an opioid order from the physician.
    c. assess the patient's pain.
    d. tell the aide to have the patient practice relaxation exercises.

58. When using charting by exception, which of the following information would need to be documented?

    a. The patient vomited after lunch.
    b. The patient's lungs are clear.
    c. The patient is eating meals well.
    d. The patient's bowels are moving daily.

59. The most malignant form of lung cancer is

    a. adenocarcinoma.
    b. large cell carcinoma.
    c. squamous cell carcinoma.
    d. small cell carcinoma (aka oat cell).

60. The Ambularm monitor should be placed on the patient's leg

    a. just below the knee.
    b. just above the knee.
    c. mid-calf.
    d. just above the ankle.

61. Which of the following should be avoided as a method of control for an older patient who has urge incontinence?

    a. Limiting fluid intake.
    b. Asking if the patient needs to urinate every two hours.
    c. Providing clothing with elasticized waistbands.
    d. Leaving the light on in the bathroom at night.

62. With the tumor, node, and metastasis (TNM) staging system for cancer, a tumor that is staged as T1, N1, and M0 means that the tumor

    a. is localized but cannot be measured.
    b. is nonmalignant.
    c. has spread to distant organs.
    d. has spread to adjacent lymph nodes.

63. Patients with celiac disease should avoid

    a. milk products.
    b. berries.
    c. gluten.
    d. soy products.

64. Which of the following ethnic groups is most sensitive to alcohol based on genetic factors?

    a. Caucasians.
    b. Native Americans.
    c. Hispanics.
    d. African-Americans.

65. If a patient states, "I tossed and turned all night," an example of paraphrasing to convey understanding is

    a. "What was upsetting you?"
    b. "You seem upset about that."
    c. "I guess you are still sleepy."
    d. "You slept poorly."

66. The component of blood that is essential for clotting is

    a. platelets.
    b. red blood cells.
    c. white blood cells.
    d. serum.

67. Most absorption of nutrients occurs in the

    a. stomach
    b. duodenum.
    c. jejunum and ileum.
    d. large intestine.

68. A patient who is nearing death has become increasingly restless. Which of the following interventions are indicated? Select all that apply.

    a. Apply restraints.
    b. Reduce sensory input (noise, sound).
    c. Speak quietly to the patient.
    d. Ask family members to leave the room.

69. Which of the following types of anemia may result from exposure to chemicals or toxins?

    a. Pernicious.
    b. Aplastic.
    c. Hemolytic.
    d. Iron deficiency.

70. The most important factor in preventing the spread of *Clostridium difficile* infection is

    a. limiting visitors.
    b. isolating infected patients.
    c. providing adequate signage.
    d. handwashing.

71. Which of the following is the best method to teach a patient to manage colostomy care after discharge?

    a. Discussion.
    b. Lecture.
    c. Demonstration/Return demonstration.
    d. Video instruction.

72. A highly inflamed and swollen pustular area that develops around a hair follicle is a

    a. furuncle.
    b. nodule.
    c. cyst.
    d. carbuncle.

73. If there is no private room available for a patient who is on contact precautions, what distance should separate the infected patient from other patients in the room?

    a. >2 feet.
    b. >3 feet.
    c. >5 feet.
    d. >6 feet.

74. Because sickle cell disease is an autosomal recessive disorder, if both parents are carriers, what percent chance does each of their offspring have of inheriting the disease?

    a. 25%.
    b. 50%.
    c. 75%.
    d. 100%.

75. Which of the following is a risk factor for the development of bladder cancer?

    a. High-protein diet.
    b. Alcohol abuse.
    c. Tobacco use.
    d. Use of illicit drugs.

76. The five risk factors that the Norton scale assesses are (1) physical condition, (2) mental state, (3) activity, (4) mobility, and (5)_____:

    a. pain.
    b. nutritional status.
    c. socioeconomic status.
    d. incontinence.

77. A patient who is near death from cancer repeatedly tells the nurse, "I'm going to get better and go home." The most appropriate response is

    a. "That would be wonderful."
    b. "That's not possible."
    c. "You are dying."
    d. "Miracles sometimes happen."

78. Which of the following is a common finding with right-sided heart failure?

    a. Dyspnea on exertion.
    b. Pitting peripheral edema.
    c. Paroxysmal nocturnal dyspnea.
    d. Cough with frothy sputum.

79. When teaching a patient to do pursed-lip breathing exercises, the target inhalation to exhalation time ratio should be

    a. 1:1.
    b. 1:2.
    c. 1:3.
    d. 1:4.

80. Which of the following behavioral characteristics most places a patient at a high risk of suicide?

    a. Daily functioning varies from poor to fairly good.
    b. Patient has few close friends.
    c. Patient expresses hostility toward others.
    d. Coping strategies are primarily destructive.

81. Which of the following effects does cigarette smoking have on the lungs? Select all that apply.

    a. Increased mucus production.
    b. Reduction of airway diameter.
    c. Abnormal constriction of distal alveoli.
    d. Reduction in ciliary action.

82. When auscultating the lungs, the nurse hears low-pitched coarse sounds that indicate secretions in the large airways. These types of breath sounds are called

    a. rhonchi.
    b. rales.
    c. wheezes.
    d. friction rubs.

83. When doing chest percussion and vibration to loosen secretions for a young adult with cystic fibrosis, the percussions should be done

    a. at varying speeds.
    b. with the hands flat.
    c. with the hands cupped.
    d. with as much force as possible.

84. During hand-off communication, it's important to

    a. review all routine care procedures.
    b. identify the patient's problems.
    c. describe results as "good," "fair," or "bad."
    d. describe all treatments in detail.

85. A confused older adult with no identification or information about her living situation is brought to the emergency department (ED) and left sitting alone in the waiting area. This type of elder mistreatment is categorized as

    a. physical abuse.
    b. emotional abuse.
    c. violation of personal rights.
    d. abandonment.

86. When irrigating a patient's ear to remove impacted cerumen, the nurse should hold the tip of the irrigating syringe

   a. 1 cm above ear canal.
   b. 2 cm above ear canal.
   c. at the opening of the ear canal.
   d. at least 1 cm inside the ear canal.

87. If a patient complains of dizziness and briefly loses consciousness after having blood drawn, the nurse should suspect that she has experienced

   a. postural hypotension.
   b. vasovagal reaction.
   c. cardiac abnormality.
   d. transient ischemic episode.

88. If a confused patient frequently climbs out of bed and walks the halls, the best approach is to

   a. use physical restrains
   b. use chemical restraints.
   c. apply bed/movement alarms.
   d. elevate all side rails.

89. With multiple myeloma, the primary initial sign or symptom of the disease is

   a. hemorrhage.
   b. anemia.
   c. fracture.
   d. skeletal pain.

90. If a patient is scheduled for major abdominal surgery, which preoperative instructions are needed? **Select all that apply.**

   a. Deep breathing and coughing exercises.
   b. Use of incentive spirometry.
   c. Home care following discharge.
   d. Leg and foot exercises.

91. If a patient wearing contact lenses splashes aftershave lotion into an eye, causing immediate tearing and burning, the first response should be to

   a. irrigate the eye with water.
   b. remove the contact lenses.
   c. administer pain medication.
   d. ask the patient to blink repeatedly.

92. Which type of pneumothorax is most likely to occur if a patient's chest tube becomes obstructed?

   a. Hemothorax.
   b. Closed.
   c. Open.
   d. Tension.

93. If an infection is spread by flying insects, such as mosquitoes, this method of transmission is

    a. direct.
    b. vector-borne.
    c. vehicle-borne.
    d. airborne.

94. In the postoperative period, the patient is expected to urinate within

    a. 1 to 2 hours.
    b. 3 to 5 hours.
    c. 6 to 8 hours.
    d. 9 to 12 hours.

95. One-tenth of a liter is equivalent to one

    a. deciliter.
    b. dekaliter.
    c. hectoliter.
    d. milliliter.

96. A patient has been recently diagnosed with leukemia and has been very stressed and crying. Which of the following is a problem-oriented coping strategy?

    a. The patient discusses anxieties with the nurse.
    b. The patient goes for long walks to help her relax.
    c. The patient schedules a series of massages.
    d. The patient attends education classes for cancer patients.

97. If a patient exercised for 20 minutes three days a week, 40 minutes two days a week, and 10 minutes twice a week, what is the patient's average exercise time per day? Answer rounded to the nearest whole number.

    _____ minutes.

98. If a patient is prescribed a medication that is enteric coated and it is to be administered per the patient's gastric feeding tube, the nurse should

    a. consult the physician about the medication.
    b. crush the tablet and administer.
    c. break up the tablet into small pieces and administer.
    d. ask the supervisor for advice.

99. Which of the following medication orders are written correctly? Select all that apply.

    a. Hydrocortisone topical cream 1% applied to right arm Q.D.
    b. Ambien 5 mg per os at BT.
    c. 15 units Humulin R subcut. 30 minutes before meals and at bedtime.
    d. Vitamin D3, 2,000 units each morning.

100. An older adult hospitalized after a fall has been prescribed 50 mg diphenhydramine (Benadryl) for sleep, but the nurse is concerned that this prescription is inappropriate for an older adult. The nurse should

    a. administer the medication as prescribed.
    b. verify the prescription with the physician.
    c. refuse to give the medication.
    d. consult a supervisor about the prescription.

101. The chance that a patient taking eight different medications will have a drug interaction is approximately

    a. 25%.
    b. 50%.
    c. 75%.
    d. 100%.

102. Which type of angina is associated with smoking, alcohol, and illicit stimulants?

    a. Variant (Prinzmetal's).
    b. Stable.
    c. Unstable.
    d. Atypical.

103. If a patient is prescribed 30 mL of liquid antacid twice daily but asks how many tablespoons are approximately equal to 30 mL, what should the nurse reply?

    _____ tablespoon(s).

104. If an order calls for eye ointment to be applied "OD," the nurse should administer the ointment to

    a. the eyelids only.
    b. both eyes.
    c. the left eye.
    d. the right eye.

105. Which of the following signs are characteristic of asthma? Select all that apply.

    a. Prolonged inspiration.
    b. Wheezing.
    c. Hypotension.
    d. Cough.

106. A patient has been experiencing orthostatic hypotension. Which of the patient's medications is most likely the cause?

    a. Metoprolol (Inderal)
    b. Metformin (Glucophage).
    c. An NSAID (Ibuprofen).
    d. Docusate (Colace).

107. A patient is considered hypoxic when his pulse oximetry falls below

    a. 95%.

    b. 90%.

    c. 85%.

    d. 80%.

108. If a patient has episodes of fever that persist for 48 to 72 hours alternating with episodes of normal temperatures that persist for up to two weeks, the pattern of her fever is described as

    a. sustained.

    b. intermittent.

    c. remittent.

    d. relapsing.

109. If a medication is prescribed at 0.150 mg, the equivalent dosage in micrograms is

    _____ µg.

110. Which of the following may help to alleviate mild sleep apnea? Select all that apply.

    a. Taking a sleep medication.

    b. Sleeping supine and flat.

    c. Avoiding alcohol for three to four hours before bedtime.

    d. Losing weight.

111. Which of the temperature measurement sites provides the most accurate and rapid core temperature measurement?

    a. Temporal artery.

    b. Axillary.

    c. Rectal.

    d. Oral.

112. If a patient has experienced a stroke on the right side of the brain, which of the following signs or symptoms should the nurse expect?

    a. Right-sided weakness.

    b. Depression and anxiety.

    c. Impaired speech

    d. Impulsivity and impaired judgment.

113. If a patient is receiving warfarin therapy, her international normalized ratio (INR) should generally be maintained at a range of

    a. 1.0 to 2.0.

    b. 2.0 to 3.0.

    c. 3.5 to 3.5.

    d. 3.5 to 4.5.

114. If a patient's chest tube becomes dislodged, the nurse's first action should be to

    a. evaluate the patient's respiratory status.

    b. notify the physician.

    c. apply pressure to the tube insertion site.

    d. call for assistance.

115. If a patient chooses words at random, such as "The dog sun burst moving and afterwards," what form of thought is the patient exhibiting?

    a. Word salad.
    b. Clang association.
    c. Neologism.
    d. Associative looseness.

116. If a nurse is to apply a transdermal nitroglycerin patch to a patient's skin, which of the following areas should be avoided? Select all that apply.

    a. Upper trunk.
    b. Abdomen.
    c. Upper arm.
    d. Lower arm.

117. If a patient expresses concern about managing ileostomy care after discharge, the most effective reassurance is

    a. "I'm sure you'll do fine."
    b. "Let's work on this together."
    c. "Don't worry. You're smart and capable."
    d. "It can be pretty complicated."

118. Which of the following characteristics are typical of chronic illness? Select all that apply.

    a. Stable periods alternating with exacerbations.
    b. Complete cure is rarely possible.
    c. Physical pathological changes are usually reversible.
    d. Complications are infrequent.

119. If a patient with syphilis is to receive 600,000 units of penicillin G procaine intramuscularly (IM) and the medication is available in 2-mL vials containing 1.2 million units, how many milliliters of medication must be administered?

    _____ mL.

120. Which of the following types of insulin should not be mixed with other types of insulin in the same syringe?

    a. NPH insulin.
    b. Regular insulin.
    c. Insulin glargine.
    d. Insulin glulisine.

121. Which foods are appropriate for a patient who is on the mechanically altered dysphagia diet, level 2? Select all that apply.

    a. Meat loaf.
    b. Canned pears or peaches.
    c. Fried bacon.
    d. French fried potatoes.

122. In an adult female, the center of gravity is usually approximately

    a. at the waist.
    b. midway between the umbilicus and symphysis pubis.
    c. at the base of the sternum.
    d. at the widest part of the hips.

123. A patient with diabetes mellitus, type 1, took insulin before lunch but ate little because of nausea. Shortly thereafter, the patient became shaky, anxious, pale, diaphoretic, combative, and confused. The immediate response should be to

    a. administer quick-acting carbohydrate.
    b. do point-of-care blood glucose.
    c. take vital signs.
    d. administer insulin.

124. A crisis is most likely to occur when a patient

    a. experiences a new or unfamiliar situation.
    b. is physically weak and tired.
    c. has inadequate coping strategies for a stressful event.
    d. lacks an adequate support system.

125. Which of the following are common opportunistic infections associated with human immunodeficiency virus/acquired immunodeficiency syndrome (HIV/AIDS)? Select all that apply.

    a. Lyme disease.
    b. Tuberculosis.
    c. Cytomegalovirus.
    d. Herpes zoster (shingles).

126. If a patient has dysphagia and is at risk for aspiration, how long should she remain sitting upright after finishing a meal?

    a. 5 to 10 minutes.
    b. 10 to 20 minutes.
    c. 20 to 30 minutes.
    d. 30 to 60 minutes.

127. Which of the following respiration patterns is characterized by two or three abnormally shallow respirations alternating with irregular periods of apnea resulting injury to the pons area of the brain?

    a. Kussmaul.
    b. Biot.
    c. Cheyne-Stokes.
    d. Bradypnea.

128. With Raynaud's disease, the patient should be advised to avoid

    a. smoking.
    b. hot weather.
    c. alcohol.
    d. milk products.

129. Which of the following antihistamines has the highest level of sedation?

    a. Fexofenadine (Allegra).
    b. Loratadine (Claritin).
    c. Diphenhydramine (Benadryl).
    d. Chlorpheniramine (Chlor-Trimeton).

130. After going to bed at night, a patient should be able to transition from awake to asleep within

    a. 5 to 10 minutes.
    b. 10 to 20 minutes.
    c. 20 to 30 minutes.
    d. 30 to 40 minutes.

131. When assisting a patient with a bed bath with soap and water, the maximum temperature of the bath water should be

    a. 90° to 100° F (32° to 37.7° C).
    b. 100° to 105° F (37.7° to 40.5° C).
    c. 110° to 115° F (43° to 46° C).
    d. 120° to 125° F (49° to 51.6° C).

132. When applying a condom sheath to a male patient, how much space should be maintained between the tip of the glans penis and the end of the condom sheath?

    a. 2.5 to 5 cm.
    b. 2 to 3 cm.
    c. 1 to 2 cm.
    d. None, the sheath should fit snugly.

133. If a patient's right leg is to be positioned in abduction, this means that the best method is to

    a. advise the patient to keep his legs apart.
    b. place a pillow or bolster between his legs.
    c. place a pillow under his right leg.
    d. cross the right ankle over his left leg.

134. If a patient's blood pressure reading is typically about 135/85, her blood pressure would be categorized as

    a. normal.
    b. prehypertension.
    c. stage 1 hypertension.
    d. stage 2 hypertension.

135. Xanthine derivatives, such as theophylline, are primarily used to treat

    a. bronchoconstriction.
    b. nasal congestion.
    c. cough.
    d. allergic reactions.

136. Patients who are unconscious should receive oral care routinely every

    a. hour.
    b. two hours.
    c. four hours.
    d. eight hours.

137. If a patient has experienced an overdose of oxycodone (OxyContin), the antidote is

    a. glucagon.
    b. N-acetylcysteine.
    c. flumazenil (Romazicon).
    d. naloxone (Narcan).

138. According to Freud, at which stage of development is masturbation and sexual relationships with peers a normal part of development?

    a. Anal stage.
    b. Phallic stage.
    c. Latency stage.
    d. Genital stage.

139. Which phase of healing occurs within minutes of injury and results in vasoconstriction?

    a. Maturation/Remodeling.
    b. Hemostasis.
    c. Proliferation.
    d. Resolution.

140. If a patient is angry with his or her physician and lashes out at the nurse, the defense mechanism that the patient is exhibiting is

    a. compensation.
    b. reaction formation.
    c. displacement.
    d. projection.

141. Possible indications of deep vein thrombosis (DVT) in the leg include which of the following? **Select all that apply.**

    a. Aching/Throbbing pain.
    b. Pallor.
    c. Vasoconstriction.
    d. Positive Homans' sign.

142. The three parameters that are evaluated with the Glasgow Coma Scale (GCS) are

    a. respirations, behavior, and appearance.
    b. response, memory, and movement.
    c. movement, reflex, and cognition.
    d. eye opening, verbal, and motor.

143. A patient who has been diagnosed with human immunodeficiency virus/acquired immunodeficiency syndrome (HIV/AIDS) has become very withdrawn and depressed, telling the nurse that she knows she is going to die. The most appropriate response for the nurse is to

    a. encourage the patient to express her feelings.
    b. remind the patient that many treatments are available.
    c. tell the patient that her feelings of depression will pass.
    d. ask the physician to refer the patient to a psychiatrist.

144. Which type of maladaptive grief response is a patient exhibiting if the patient remains fixed in the anger stage of grieving, refusing to cooperate and insulting family and healthcare providers?

    a. Prolonged.
    b. Distorted.
    c. Delayed.
    d. Inhibited.

145. If a patient engages in moderate aerobic exercise, such as brisk walking, how much time per week should she plan to exercise to meet recommended exercise guidelines for healthy adults?

    a. 75 minutes.
    b. 100 minutes.
    c. 150 minutes.
    d. 175 minutes.

146. Keyboards and monitors are in each patient's room so that documentation can be done at the point of care, and the monitor is mounted on the wall. When viewing the monitor, the nurse should adjust the monitor so that the top of the monitor is

    a. at or slightly below the level of the eyes.
    b. at or slightly above the level of the eyes.
    c. placed so the eyes are centered midmonitor.
    d. in line with the bottom of the viewer's chin.

147. What percentage of the body weight is accounted for by water?

    a. 20% to 30%.
    b. 30% to 40%.
    c. 40% to 50%.
    d. 50% to 60%.

148. A patient's nosebleed has stopped, but the nurse notes that the patient is swallowing frequently. The nurse should suspect that

    a. the patient is nervous and anxious.
    b. blood is running down the patient's throat.
    c. the patient is dehydrated and thirsty.
    d. the patient's throat is irritated.

149. The movement of water between two compartments separated by a semipermeable membrane is referred to as

    a. active transport.
    b. diffusion.
    c. osmosis.
    d. facilitated diffusion.

150. At what degree of angle should a subcutaneous injection be administered?

   a. 45 to 90.
   b. 90.
   c. 30 to 45.
   d. 30.

151. The normal value for potassium (K+) is

   a. 2.0 to 2.5 mEq/L.
   b. 3.0 to 3.5 mEq/L.
   c. 3.5 to 5.5 mEq/L.
   d. 5.5 to 7.5 mEq/L.

152. Which of the following is an indication that a nurse has breached a professional boundary?

   a. The nurse gives a birthday card to a long-term patient.
   b. The nurse likes one patient more than another.
   c. The nurse sits with the patient when the patient receives bad news.
   d. The nurse tells the patient a personal secret.

153. If a hospitalized patient requests that a tribal healer participate in his treatment, the nurse should

   a. tell the patient that is not acceptable.
   b. help to arrange for this to happen.
   c. advise the patient to wait until after discharge.
   d. ask the patient why he wants a tribal healer.

154. For which of the following sexually transmitted diseases is no cure yet available?

   a. Genital herpes simplex virus, type 1 or 2 (HSV-1 or HSV-2).
   b. Gonorrhea.
   c. Chlamydia.
   d. Syphilis.

155. If a patient with obesity has begun a weight reduction program, a reasonable weekly weight loss is

   a. 5 to 6 pounds.
   b. 3 to 4 pounds.
   c. 1 to 2 pounds.
   d. 1/2 to 1 pound.

156. According to Maslow's hierarchy of needs, which need must be met first?

   a. Need for self-actualization.
   b. Physiological needs.
   c. Need for safety and security.
   d. Belonging/Love needs.

157. Which of the following are characteristics of early adulthood (about ages 20 to 40)? **Select all that apply.**

   a. Satisfaction with life/career.
   b. Establishment of personal/economic independence.
   c. Stability.
   d. Experimentation.

158. With conscious sedation, the patient is

   a. awake but has no later memory of the procedure.
   b. awake and has only vague and fleeting memories of the procedure.
   c. awake and alert throughout the procedure.
   d. completely unconscious throughout the procedure.

159. After giving a patient an injection, the nurse should

   a. wrap the syringe and needle in paper before discarding.
   b. bend or break the needle before discarding.
   c. discard the syringe and needle intact.
   d. recap the needle before discarding.

160. When carrying out cardiopulmonary resuscitation (CPR), the cardiac compression rate per minute should be

   a. 40.
   b. 60.
   c. 80.
   d. 100.

161. Which of the following are characteristic changes found in the gastrointestinal system of older adults? **Select all that apply.**

   a. Decreased production of saliva.
   b. Increased motility of esophagus.
   c. More rapid gastric emptying.
   d. Impaired intestinal absorption of fats and nutrients.

162. Which of the following are important steps in fall prevention for older adults? **Select all that apply.**

   a. Balance and exercise programs.
   b. Vision and hearing checkups.
   c. Limit activities.
   d. Keep environment safe.

163. Which of the following foods is an example of a "starchy" (high-carbohydrate) vegetable?

   a. Corn.
   b. Carrots.
   c. Asparagus.
   d. Spinach.

164. A patient tells the nurse that he has a question about the DASH diet that the nutritionist reviewed with him. Which of the following is the best response?

    a. "I'll tell the nutritionist that you still have some questions."
    b. "Ask your doctor about that question."
    c. "The answer is probably in your diet handout."
    d. "Ask me. If I don't know the answer, I'll get the information for you."

165. Which of the following is an example of secondary prevention?

    a. Routine Pap smear.
    b. Exercise program.
    c. Smoking cessation.
    d. 12-step program.

166. When a patient's respiratory status must be continually monitored, the most effective method is to rely on

    a. visual observation.
    b. pulse oximetry.
    c. auscultation.
    d. patient's complaint of dyspnea.

167. The study of actions that are considered right or wrong when related to medicine, treatment, life, or death is

    a. morality.
    b. ethics.
    c. bioethics.
    d. values.

168. A disinfectant that is bacteriostatic

    a. spreads some types of bacteria.
    b. destroys bacterial spores.
    c. destroys bacteria.
    d. prevents growth and reproduction of some bacteria.

169. The moral principle that decrees that the nurse provide equal care and attention to all patients is

    a. beneficence.
    b. nonmaleficence.
    c. justice.
    d. fidelity.

170. If a nurse takes a photograph of a patient to use in a journal article without the patient's consent, this is an example of

    a. negligence.
    b. invasion of privacy.
    c. malpractice.
    d. unprofessional conduct.

171. Items that belong to a patient should not be placed on the floor primarily because

    a. the floor is considered grossly contaminated.
    b. the item may contaminate the floor.
    c. bending over to pick up the item may cause back injury.
    d. the items may be overlooked and lost or misplaced.

172. If a nurse provides emergent care at the scene of an accident but the person dies from severe injuries, the nurse

    a. may be legally liable for the person's death.
    b. is protected by federal Good Samaritan law.
    c. is protected by state Good Samaritan law.
    d. should have provided no care without informed consent.

173. If a patient has been placed in physical restraints to protect the safety of himself and others, what is the maximum number of consecutive hours that the patient may generally be maintained in restraints with renewal of orders?

    a. 4 hours.
    b. 8 hours.
    c. 12 hours.
    d. 24 hours.

174. When removing a mask secured with two ties, the nurse should first

    a. untie the lower tie.
    b. untie the upper tie.
    c. untie either tie.
    d. leave the ties intact and pull the mask up over the head.

175. If a female patient's waist measurement is 37 inches and her hip measurement is 44 inches, what is the patient's waist-to-hip ratio? **Record to two decimal places.**

    _____.

176. If the nurse is aspirating stomach contents per an NG tube to ensure proper placement before administering a tube feeding, the pH reading that likely indicates gastric fluid is

    a. 4.0
    b. 7.6
    c. 7.38
    d. 7.10

177. If a patient complains of rectal discomfort, abdominal distention, and flatus as well as a continuous urge to defecate and states he has passed only small amounts of liquid stool for the past three to four days, the nurse should suspect

    a. bowel obstruction.
    b. diarrhea.
    c. constipation.
    d. fecal impaction.

178. If a female patient objects to a male nurse administering a vaginal suppository, the nurse should

    a. instruct the patient in self-administration.
    b. discard the suppository and document patient's refusal.
    c. arrange for a female nurse to administer the suppository.
    d. remind the patient that many doctors are male.

179. If the nurse has asked an unlicensed assistive personnel (UAP) to assist a patient with mouth care and walks by the open door to the room 30 minutes later and notes that the UAP is assisting the patient to brush his teeth, the nurse's greatest concern should be that

    a. the door is open.
    b. the patient is compliant.
    c. the mouth care was delayed.
    d. the care be documented.

180. During manual removal of a fecal impaction, the patient becomes very faint with a sudden drop in blood pressure and heart rate. The most likely cause is

    a. heart attack.
    b. vasovagal response.
    c. rectal perforation.
    d. stroke.

181. Which of the following types of laxatives/cathartics is most recommended for chronic constipation?

    a. Stimulant.
    b. Lubricant.
    c. Emollient/wetting.
    d. Bulk-forming.

182. If a patient's hand is swelling and a ring is beginning to impair circulation, the first method to use in attempting to remove the ring is

    a. twisting ring downward to attempt removal without further intervention.
    b. elevating and soaking hand in cool water and applying lubricant before attempting removal.
    c. using the string-wrap method with a tape anchor.
    d. using a circular-blade ring cutter to cut the ring off the finger.

183. Following a vasectomy, which comment by the patient indicates a need for education?

    a. "I know that sterility is almost immediate after vasectomy."
    b. "I need to have semen analysis in about 12 weeks."
    c. "Vasectomy does not increase the risk of testicular cancer."
    d. "I should avoid ejaculating for one week."

184. Which of the following observations may indicate that a patient with cognitive impairment and the inability to verbalize pain is experiencing pain?

    a. Patient is sleeping frequently.
    b. Patient's respiration rate has slowed.
    c. Patient is tense and combative and appears frightened.
    d. Patient's blood pressure and heart rate have decreased.

Answers and Explanations

1. D: If a patient with a history of asthma is experiencing an acute exacerbation with wheezing and dyspnea, the medication likely to provide the most immediate relief is albuterol, which is a beta-adrenergic agonist, commonly used during the acute stage of asthma, because this class of drugs provides fast-acting bronchodilation. Because these drugs have some vasoconstrictive properties, they should be avoided in patients with uncontrolled cardiac dysrhythmias and high stroke risk.

2. B: Patients with gynoid (pear-shaped) obesity have increased risk of varicose veins, cellulitis, osteoporosis, and increased triglycerides. However, gynoid obesity poses less of a risk to overall health than android (apple-shaped) obesity, which is implicated in diabetes and heart disease as well as breast and endometrial cancer. With gynoid obesity, most of the excess weight is carried in the upper arms, buttocks, and thighs.

3. C: Prolonged immobilization is one of the primary risk factors for the development of pulmonary embolus in the postoperative period because immobilization can lead to deep vein thrombosis (DVT). DVT, in turn, can lead to pulmonary embolus if part of the thrombus formation breaks away and enters the bloodstream. It is for this reason that patients are encouraged to move about in bed and ambulate as soon as possible. Other risk factors include hypercoagulability of the blood, which makes it prone to clot, and older age.

4. A: A patient who has undergone a colectomy for a bowel obstruction and is refusing to turn, get out of bed, or cooperate should likely be assessed for pain first because the most common reason for failing to move after surgery is pain. Next, the wound should be examined, vital signs taken, and emotional status evaluated. The patient may be fearful that movement will increase pain or cause the wound to tear or open.

5. C: If a patient has diabetic ketoacidosis and her arterial blood gases are pH, 7.22; $PaCO_2$, 41 mm Hg; and HCO_3, 15 mEq/L, the acid-base imbalance indicated is metabolic acidosis. The patient is acidotic because her pH is less than 7.35. The $PaCO_2$ remains within normal limits, so the problem is not respiratory, but the HCO_3 is low at 15 mEq/L (normal 22–26 mEq/L), indicating a metabolic abnormality. The condition is uncompensated because the $PaCO_2$ has not changed to compensate.

6. B: If an Orthodox Jewish patient who is refusing to use electrical appliances on the Sabbath will not use the call bell or respond to the intercom, the nurse should provide him with a hand bell or alternate means of calling the nurse. The nurse should not try to pressure the patient into changing religious practice and should make an effort to look in on him whenever possible, although every 15 to 30 minutes may not be possible.

7. A: In the communication process, *channel* refers to the means of sending and receiving a message through visual, auditory, or tactile senses, and it includes not only the voice but also facial expression. The communication process includes the referent (motivator), the sender, the receiver, the message, the channel, the feedback (return message), interpersonal variables (influencing factors), and the environment (setting for the interaction).

8. 45 mg: If a patient with kidney disease is limited to 0.6 mg protein per kg of body weight and she weighs 165 pounds, she is allowed 45 mg of protein daily. The first step is to convert pounds to kilograms:

$$165/2.2 = 75.$$

Then 75 is multiplied by 0.6 (the protein allowance per kg):

75 x 0.6 = 45 mg protein.

9. C: Prolonged antibiotic or corticosteroid use increases the risk of candidiasis, most commonly caused by *Candida albicans*. Candidiasis can occur in the mouth (thrush), skin (cutaneous), or vagina (yeast infection). *Candida* can also invade the bloodstream and result in systemic infection or infections of various organs. Oral infections are usually treated with nystatin or amphotericin B oral suspensions or buccal tablets. Treatment varies according to the anatomic site of the infection.

10. D: The correct position to place a patient in when he is going into shock is Trendelenburg (feet elevated above the heart). If the patient is not on a bed that can be placed in this position, then he should lie flat with pillows placed under his legs to elevate them. Although treatment varies somewhat depending on the cause and type of shock, in most cases, fluid resuscitation with intravenous (IV) fluids is necessary as well as administration of medication such as dopamine to constrict blood vessels and increase blood pressure.

11. B: Empathy is the ability of the nurse to listen to a patient, perceive the patient's feelings, and understand the patient's perspectives. Sympathy, on the other hand, involves feelings of pity or concern for the patient. Sympathy, a subjective response, can sometimes interfere with objective evaluation. Patience is the ability to deal with problems without getting upset or angry. Compassion is a feeling of understanding that can move a person to action in response.

12. A: The laboratory test value that the nurse should report to the physician because it is outside of the normal range is hemoglobin 9.1 g/dL. Hemoglobin carries oxygen and is decreased in anemia and increased in polycythemia. Normal values vary somewhat by gender and include

- Males >18 years: 14.0–17.46 g/dL and
- Females >18 years: 12.0–16.0 g/dL.

Hemoglobin is generally reported with hematocrit, which shows the proportion of red blood cells in a liter of blood and usually is about three times the hemoglobin number:

- Males >18 years: 45–52% and
- Females >18 years: 36–48%.

13. C: If the nurse administers a medication to the wrong patient, her response should be to assess the patient for an adverse reaction. The nurse should also check the patient's known allergies. Then, the nurse should notify the physician and the supervisor. The medication should be documented in the patient's health record, but the incident report detailing the error is filed separately.

14. B: The electrolyte imbalance that is likely to occur with persistent vomiting and diarrhea is hyponatremia. Gastric and intestinal fluids contain high levels of sodium, so sodium can become depleted with nausea and diarrhea. Hyponatremia is a sodium level of less than 135 mEq/L. This type of hyponatremia resulting from hypovolemia is characterized by dry mucous membranes, orthostatic hypotension, tachycardia, and poor skin turgor. The patient may appear weak, stuporous, confused, and/or lethargic.

15. D: If a patient is declared brain dead after a motorcycle accident, a person who is specially trained, often a transplant coordinator or other designated healthcare professional, should discuss organ donation with the family. However, the nurse should remain supportive of the family, answer any questions, and ensure that the transplant coordinator or designated professional is notified in advance. This is often a very emotional time for family members, so it's important that only people who are trained approach the family about organ donation.

16. C and D: The elbow is a hinge joint and only has two motions: flexion and extension. With flexion, the elbow bends so that the forearm moves toward the shoulder and the hand is level with the shoulder. The range of motion is 150 degrees, involving primarily the biceps brachii, brachialis, and brachioradialis muscles. With extension, the elbow and arm straighten. The range of motion is also 150 degrees, but extension involves primarily the triceps brachii muscles.

17. C: According to Erikson, the primary task of young adults is intimacy versus isolation. The young adult should have developed a sense of identity and should be prepared to love others and establish intimate relationships. If the young adult experiences disappointment or rejection in efforts to establish intimacy, then isolation may result as the person withdraws from others. Young adults who are ill or undergoing periods of stress may have an increased need of intimacy and the support of others.

18. D: Watery wound drainage that is yellow tinged and has occasional red streaks would be categorized as serosanguineous. Serous drainage, which is essentially serum, is watery and clear and often slightly yellow tinged. Sanguineous drainage is thicker and frankly bloody. Purulent discharge is thick and opaque and may have a foul odor, depending on the type of infection that is present. When describing discharge, the nurse should note the color, consistency, odor, and estimated volume.

19. B: The response that is most helpful if a patient who has been awaiting chemotherapy treatment suddenly becomes anxious and exhibits rapid pulse, trembling, and diaphoresis is "What were you thinking about right before you started feeling bad?" This encourages the patient to focus less on the physical reactions and more on feelings and to discuss the source of anxiety. Admonitions to stop worrying are usually not helpful, although some patients may benefit from deep breathing and relaxation especially if they have practiced the technique as a way to reduce stress.

20. A and B: The religions that specifically forbid the eating of pork are Judaism and Islam. Although many Hindus avoid eating pork, this is a cultural practice rather than religious because pigs are considered by many Hindus to be unclean because they eat garbage and cool themselves in the mud. However, the nurse should never make assumptions about a patient's religious practices even though they have listed a preference for a specific religion. People may identify with a religion while not maintaining dietary restrictions or religious rituals.

21. A: If a patient is very upset because she is nearing her 65th birthday, the type of crisis the patient is likely experiencing is life transitional. Life transitions are those changes in life that are predictable (graduation from high school, marriage, aging, divorce, moving) but over which the patient may feel a lack of control and may be unsure as to how to deal with the changes brought about by the transition, even if it is ultimately positive.

22. C: Oropharyngeal suctioning is indicated for a patient who has had a stroke with right-sided paralysis and has persistent drooling and impaired swallowing. This type is the least invasive and uncomfortable for the patient and uses a Yankauer nozzle to suction mucous secretions from the mouth in order to prevent the patient from aspirating them. Patients should be placed in the semi-Fowler's or upright position for suctioning.

23. B: If a patient is allowed no weight bearing on the left leg, the most appropriate crutch gait is three-point. With this gait, all of the weight is borne on the crutches at the onset. The uninvolved leg moves forward and then bears all the weight while the person advances both crutches. The left leg is usually maintained in a slightly flexed position, or, if that isn't possible, it is extended slightly in front.

24. D: If a patient develops signs of bacterial food poisoning within 30 minutes of eating, the most likely causative agent is *Staphylococcus aureus. Staphylococcus* infections occur much more rapidly than other types of food poisoning, although the symptoms may be delayed for up to 7 hours in some patients. Symptoms are usually nausea, vomiting, and diarrhea. Treatment includes supportive care, electrolyte replacement if needed, and antiemetics.

25. B: Adults should receive the tetanus, diphtheria, and pertussis (Tdap) vaccination one time. Then, every 10 years the patient should have the Td booster, which serves as a booster for tetanus and diphtheria, but not pertussis. Tdap is usually given at age 11 or 12, but adults who did not receive this vaccination should do so as soon as possible. Women who are pregnant should also receive the Tdap vaccination in order to provide protection from pertussis for the neonate.

26. A: The cultural/ethnic group that is likely to experience a condition referred to as "ghost sickness," which may involve having bad dreams or exhibiting abnormal behavior, is the Navajo as well as a few other tribes. The Navajo believe that ghost sickness is caused by evil spirits and treatment requires overcoming this spirit through a healing ritual. Patients may be terrified and complain of weakness and loss of appetite. Patients often believe that one particular deceased person is causing the problem because the person was not properly buried or cared for after death.

27. C: In order to prevent food poisoning, ground beef should be cooked to 160° F. Ground beef should not be served rare because it is more likely to be contaminated because the grinding process mixes the bacteria throughout the meat whereas solid pieces of meat have surface contamination that is more easily destroyed in cooking. Poultry should also always be cooked well done and to a minimum of 165° F, although many authorities recommend cooking to 180° F.

28. A and **D:** If a patient has nonblanching erythema of intact skin over the coccygeal area, this is a stage 1 pressure ulcer. Treatments that may be indicated include frequent turning and positioning the patient to avoid pressure on the reddened area. A transparent dressing may be applied to protect the skin as well. Pressure-reducing devices, such as foam overlays, are indicated. The patient should be kept clean and dry with adequate nutrition and fluid intake.

29. D: Peak flow meters measure the highest airflow during forced exhalation. Peak flow is usually monitored for patients with moderate to severe asthma because it can help to determine when airflow is impaired. Typically, the meters are set for each individual, with a green range that indicates the patient is doing well, a yellow range that indicates airflow has decreased and the patient may need intervention, and a red range that indicates the patient is in an emergent situation and needs immediate medical attention.

30. C: If a patient has slipped down in the bed and is in an uncomfortable position, the nursing action that should be avoided is to grasp the patient under the arms from the head of the bed and pull. This is not only uncomfortable for the patient and increases the risk of friction damage to the skin but also increases the risk of back injury to the nurse. Various methods can be used to move the patient, including the use of a slip sheet or trapeze.

31. B: Fistulas are a common complication of Crohn's disease. Fistulas may develop between layers of intestines or between intestines and the bladder or the vagina. Crohn's disease is one type of inflammatory bowel disease. Crohn's disease can affect any part of the gastrointestinal system, although it is most common in the terminal ileum and the colon. Deep ulcerations develop, and scarring can form strictures that result in bowel obstruction. Other common complications include diarrhea, fever, rectal bleeding, and perforation.

32. D: The complementary therapy that uses meters and monitors to help patients learn to control bodily functions is biofeedback. Biofeedback involves a number of different techniques, but all methods provide feedback of some type to help the patient gauge the effectiveness of their actions. For example, a patient may concentrate on relaxing and reducing the heart rate while watching a heart rate monitor. Over time, the patient should be able to slow the heart without the feedback. Biofeedback is often used to help control hypertension, pain, and headaches.

33. A: If a patient complains that something in the abdominal surgical site "gave way" when coughing and the dressings are immediately saturated with serosanguineous drainage, the nurse should suspect dehiscence. The patient should be positioned in a supine position with the knees slightly flexed to reduce tension on the incision. The wound should be examined to verify the dehiscence and determine its extent, and the physician should be notified. The patient should be reassured and administered pain medication if it is due.

34. C: If the nurse is assigned by the supervisor to do a task for which he does not feel prepared, then he should tell his supervisor immediately so that the task can be delegated to someone else or he can receive instruction or assistance in carrying out the task. The nurse should never attempt to carry out a task without adequate knowledge and/or experience because this can result in medical errors or injury to the patient.

35. B: If a confused patient insists that someone is being tortured when she hears the ambulance siren, the best response is "That noise is an ambulance siren." The nurse should orient the patient to reality by saying what is true without arguing with the patient ("No one is being tortured here") or playing along with the patient's delusion ("Don't worry; I'll take care of it"). Stating, "No one is going to hurt you. You are safe," does not really address the issue that is confusing the patient—the sound of the siren.

36. 195 mg: If a patient weighs 143 pounds and must receive a medication at the rate of 3 mg/kg, the patient should receive 195 mg. The first step is to convert pounds to kilograms: 143/2.2 = 65. The patient weighs 65 kg, so the next step is to multiply 65 by 3 (because the required dosing is 3mg/kg) to determine the needed dosage: 65 X 3 = 195.

37. D: If a patient has an ascending colostomy, the consistency of the stool is usually liquid because most absorption of fluids takes place within the colon. A patient with an ascending colostomy will not need to do colostomy irrigations but will need to continually wear a colostomy appliance, so this may be very stressful for patients, especially in the beginning when they are learning self-management. A number of different types of appliances are available.

38. C: For nasopharyngeal suctioning of adults, the catheter should be inserted approximately 16 cm (about 6.5 inches). The nurse should be careful to apply no suction while the catheter is inserted because this may result in damage to the mucous membranes. The catheter should only be inserted on inhalation, and the patient should be cautioned to avoid swallowing, which increases the risk that the tube will enter the esophagus.

39. A: If a patient has severe ascites (most often associated with cirrhosis or liver cancer), a paracentesis is usually done only to relieve severe dyspnea or pain because the fluid rapidly accumulates again, and the procedure may increase the loss of electrolytes. If a patient is to undergo paracentesis, she must empty her bladder first. Ideally, the patient should have the procedure while sitting upright because this facilitates drainage of the fluid.

40. B: If a patient is able to respond but does not recall his son's name or the date and doesn't know where he is, he could be described as disoriented. If the onset of disorientation is sudden, it may indicate a medical emergency, such as with a head injury, and the patient's vital signs should be recorded and the physician notified. In some cases, disorientation may result from medications. Patients with Alzheimer's disease are often disoriented, especially as the disease progresses.

41. D: If the nurse is caring for a patient who is receiving a transfusion of platelets because of severe thrombocytopenia, the observation that should be reported immediately is chills and itching because these symptoms may indicate a transfusion reaction. Bruising at the IV puncture site is common for those with a low platelet counts as is a slight bloody discharge when blowing the nose. Sleepiness and lethargy are unrelated to the transfusion

42. A and B: Objective data are data that can be measured or observed directly. Examples of objective data include the following:

- "BP 128/86, pulse 84" and
- "Erythema extends 2 cm around the wound perimeter."

Subjective data are data that are reported but that cannot be measured, such as "Patient complains of headache and dizziness." These symptoms are not observable externally. Although a scale is used to describe pain, such as in "Patient's pain decreased from 8 to 2 on a 1 to 10 scale," this is subjective because the measure of the scale depends on what the patient says and cannot be verified by observation.

43. C: The type of pressure-reducing bed/mattress that can result in increased perspiration and dehydration is the air-fluidized bed. Patients experience evaporative fluid loss because warm air constantly blows across the patient. The operating temperature can be set between 82 and 102° F (usually maintained between 85 and 95° F for most patients). A patient's electrolyte levels should be checked regularly and fluid intake should be monitored when the patient is using the bed. About two-thirds of the patient's body is immersed.

44. B: If a patient that the nurse is caring for has had continuous IV therapy for four days and the nurse notes that the IV insertion site in his arm is swollen and the tissue is red and tender with a red streak extending proximally, the most likely reason is phlebitis. The IV infusion should be discontinued and restarted at a different site. Mild phlebitis will usually clear without specific treatment, although antibiotics may be indicated if purulent discharge is evident.

45. D: If a patient has developed a postoperative infection and has a large open wound that must be packed with alginate, the alginate should be packed loosely because it absorbs exudate and swells into a gelled form. Alginate is made from brown seaweed and comes in various forms: wafers, rope, or fibers. Alginate can be used with wounds that have undermining and tunneling. Alginates must be covered by a secondary dressing.

46. C: If a patient who is being discharged states she is happy about going home but appears anxious, is wringing her hands (a self-comforting measure), and is avoiding eye contact (which could mean the patient is fearful or being untruthful), the most therapeutic response is "You say you're happy, but you seem anxious." This is an observational statement about what the nurse sees and how the nurse interprets it but does not directly contradict the patient.

47. B: When assisting a patient with overactive bladder to extend time between urinations, if the patient usually urinates every hour, the first goal should be to extend this time by 15 minutes. The nurse should advise the patient to try to hold urination until the scheduled time but to urinate if in

83

danger of incontinence. The patient should be urged to stop and take deep breaths rather than immediately rushing to the bathroom, which usually increases urgency.

48. A: Bariatric beds are intended for patients who are more than 100 lb. (45 kg) overweight. The bariatric bed is adjustable so that the patient can be in an upright or sitting position and the bed can be wheeled for transportation. Even though the bed is wider than the normal bed, the standard bariatric bed fits through doorways. However, full or double-wide bariatric beds are available for patients up to 1,000 lb. (450 kg), and these beds must be set up and dismantled inside a room because they cannot fit through doorways.

49. D: If a woman tells the nurse that her child has swallowed a poison, the first question should be "What poison did the child swallow?" This information is the most critical because protocols for treatment vary according to the type of poison. Once this is established, the nurse needs to ask when the incident occurred, how much poison was swallowed, and whether the child vomited because some poisons can cause additional damage if vomited before they are neutralized.

50. C: If a patient is developing pneumonia, the stage of the disease that is likely to occur first is congestion. During this early stage, the microorganisms have reached the alveoli, which causes fluid to fill the alveoli, providing a medium for the microorganisms to multiply and impairs gas exchange. The next stage is dilation of the capillaries (red hepatization), which causes the lungs to take on a red appearance as organisms, neutrophils, red blood cells, and fibrin fill the alveoli. Consolidation (gray hepatization) occurs as the leukocytes and fibrin fill the alveoli. Resolution is the healing stage when the lung tissue recovers.

51. B: In the orientation phase of a therapeutic relationship, the primary role of the nurse is to build trust and to begin to help the patient to set goals. This phase begins when the nurse meets the patient for the first time. The patient may be reluctant to admit to the need for help until she feels more comfortable with the nurse, so the nurse may spend some time engaging in nonthreatening conversation to put the patient at ease before beginning to clarify the problems and to outline patient and nurse obligations.

52. A: The wound care product that is designed to hydrate a wound is hydrogel, which is a glycerin- or water-based product. Hydrogel is applied directly to partial- or full-thickness wounds that are dry or have only a small amount of exudate in order to provide moisture and autolysis. Hydrogel should not be used on third-degree burns or wounds with heavy exudate because it has limited absorbent quality. Hydrogel can cause skin maceration and candidiasis of the periwound area. Some products have adhesive covers, so they can be left in place for two or three days.

53. D: The primary problem with narrative documentation is that it's difficult to retrieve data because important details may be embedded in a long narrative description. The reader may need to read through many days of narratives to determine if patterns are emerging in the patient's condition. Narrative documentation can be quite time consuming and may vary widely in quality. It is often repetitive, with the same information about routine care (such as "mouth care") repeated many times.

54. C: When using the PLISSIT assessment of sexuality, the nurse should always begin the assessment by asking permission to discuss sexual matters:

- (P) Permission
- (L) (I) Limited information: Related to sexual health problems that the patient is experiencing.

- (S) (S) Specific suggestions: May be provided if the nurse is clear about the problem.
- (T) Intensive therapy: Referral to the appropriate healthcare professional as indicated.

55. 12 m: If a patient is to receive 600 mg of cephalexin oral suspension per NG tube every six hours, and the oral suspension contains 250 mg per 5 mL, the nurse should administer 12 mL for each dose. The formula:

- mg needed/mg available × volume.
- 600/250 = 2.4 × 5 = 12 mL.

56. B: Patients with cirrhosis of the liver should be advised that they must maintain abstinence of alcohol. Patients should also be advised to avoid the use of aspirin or nonsteroidal anti-inflammatory drugs (NSAIDs) because of the increased risk of bleeding. There is no treatment that can reverse cirrhosis, so treatment usually focuses on maintenance and prevention of ascites and includes rest, vitamin B-complex vitamins, a low-sodium diet, and diuretics. Paracentesis may be done to relieve severe dyspnea or pain associated with ascites.

57. C: If an aide reports to the nurse that a patient with pancreatic cancer is complaining of severe abdominal pain and lying rigidly in bed and he has only an NSAID ordered for pain, the nurse's first action should be to assess the patient's pain because she should not administer pain medication based on someone else's assessment. If the patient's pain is severe, then the NSAID may be inadequate, so the nurse may need to contact the physician for a stronger analgesic.

58. A: When using charting by exception, the information that would need to be documented is the following: The patient vomited after lunch. With charting by exception, a baseline is established for the patient, and as long as the patient stays within that baseline (such as having clear lungs, eating well, and having daily bowel movements), then no further notation needs to be done about those matters. However, vomiting is an abnormal finding and would, therefore, need to be documented.

59. D: The most malignant form of lung cancer is small cell carcinoma (aka oat cell carcinoma), which causes about 10% to 15% of lung cancers. Small cell carcinoma tends to spread early and quickly and responds poorly to treatment. Almost all cases of small cell carcinoma are associated with cigarette smoking or exposure to environmental carcinogens. Current treatments are usually not curative, and patients may be encouraged to participate in clinical trials in an effort to prolong life.

60. B: The Ambularm should be placed on the patient's leg just above the knee. The nurse should measure the mid-calf area to determine the correct cuff size. A small battery is snapped into place on the side of the cuff to activate the alarm. The alarm sounds when the sensor detects a near-vertical position, so patients need to keep their leg in a fairly horizontal position. Patients who are kicking their legs about or extremely restless may not be good candidates for this alarm.

61. A: If an older patient has urge incontinence, limiting fluid intake is a poor strategy because dehydration is common in older adults, and concentrated urine may increase bladder irritability, making incontinence worse. Most adults require about eight glasses of water daily. However, if the patient's fluid intake is adequate, the patient may be discouraged from drinking large amounts of liquids in the evening before retiring because this will likely result in nocturia, increasing the risk of incontinence.

62. D: With the TNM staging system for cancer, a tumor that is staged as T1, N1, and M0 means that the tumor is stage 1, so it is localized. N1 means that it has spread to one or more adjacent lymph nodes. M0 means that there is no metastasis. The TNM staging system is useful for a number of different types of cancers. T refers to the primary tumor, N to nodes, and M to metastasis. Numbers indicate the degree of severity from 1 to 4. A zero indicates absence. X indicates that the component cannot be measured or evaluated.

63. C: Patients with celiac disease should avoid gluten, which is found in grains such as wheat, rye, oats, and barley. Gluten is also commonly found in many prepared foods, including prepared meats and salad dressings. Even a very small amount of gluten can result in severe diarrhea and steatorrhea. The only adequate treatment for celiac disease is complete elimination of gluten from the diet. Many gluten-free products, including breads and pastries, are now available.

64. B: Native Americans are especially sensitive to alcohol based on genetic factors. They have faster metabolism of alcohol than other ethnic groups and less tolerance. Rates of fetal alcohol syndrome are highest among Native Americans. About 12% of deaths among Native Americans are attributed to alcohol. Native Americans are about two and a half times more likely to have chronic liver disease than Caucasians because of alcohol intake.

65. D: If a patient states, "I tossed and turned all night," an example of paraphrasing to convey understanding is "You slept poorly." Paraphrasing restates in simpler words what the patient has stated rather than making any kind of judgment about meaning. When a nurse paraphrases something the patient has said, this is an effective method of conveying to the patient that the nurse is listening to the patient and understanding the patient's message.

66. A: The component of blood that is essential for clotting is platelets (thrombocytes). Platelets are the smallest component of the blood because they are fragments of a large cell (megakaryocytes) rather than a complete cell like the other blood cells, so platelets have no nucleus. Platelets are produced in the bone marrow and then leave and circulate in the blood. Platelets are disk shaped in their resting state but develop a globular shape with pseudopodia (false feet) so they can adhere to each other when activated to form a clot.

67. C: Most absorption of nutrients occurs in the small intestine, in the jejunum and ileum. The digestive process starts in the mouth as saliva and chewing begin to break down the food that then enters the esophagus and travels to the stomach, where the food is further mixed and broken down by the addition of acid and enzymes. This process continues in the duodenum with most absorption of nutrients occurring in the small intestine. Fluid continues to be absorbed in the large intestine.

68. B and C: If a patient who is nearing death has become increasingly restless, the nurse should try to reduce sensory input (noise and sound) and speak quietly to the patient in a soothing voice. If restlessness is associated with pain, then the patient may need analgesia. Restraints should not be applied, although the side rails should be up and padded if the patient is flailing his arms or legs. Family members should not be asked to leave the room.

69. B: Aplastic anemia may result from exposure to chemicals or toxins, which interferes with the bone marrow's ability to produce cells, so it can affect all elements of the blood, including red blood cells. Symptoms depend on the severity and may include weakness, fatigue, dyspnea, headache, pallor, tachycardia, heart failure, ecchymoses, petechiae, hemorrhage, and infection. Treatment focuses on identifying and eliminating the cause and transfusions of necessary blood components. For severe cases, bone marrow transplantation is the treatment of choice.

70. D: The most important factor in preventing the spread of *Clostridium difficile* infection is handwashing. The pathogens are spread in the feces, most often when the hands of healthcare providers come in contact with contaminated environmental surfaces. Because infection with *C. difficile* often results in watery diarrhea and may cause incontinence, contamination can easily occur, so washing the hands thoroughly with soap and water is essential because spores might not be killed with alcohol rubs.

71. C: The best method to teach a patient to manage colostomy care after discharge is to provide a demonstration and have the patient do a return demonstration. Although supportive materials, such as handouts, guidelines, and videos, may help to prepare the patient or reinforce knowledge, knowing and doing are two different things. Because the patient must carry out a process with numerous steps, the practice and demonstration of skills is critical.

72. A: A highly inflamed and swollen pustular area that develops around a hair follicle is a furuncle.

Clustered areas of multiple such lesions connected subcutaneously are referred to as carbuncles. Furuncles and carbuncles are typically caused by *Staphylococcus aureus* (common skin bacteria) or methicillin-resistant *S. aureus* (MRSA). Furuncles commonly occur on the back of the neck, the breasts, the buttocks, and the face. Furuncles are very painful and usually require incision and drainage to drain the purulent exudate and antibiotics to promote healing.

73. B: If there is no private room available for a patient who is on contact precautions, a distance of greater than three feet should separate the patient from others.

Contact	Use personal protective equipment (PPE), including gown and gloves, for all contacts with the patient or patient's immediate environment. Maintain the patient in a private room or >3 feet away from other patients.
Droplet	Use a mask while caring for the patient. Maintain the patient in a private room or >3 feet away from other patients with a curtain separating them. Use a patient mask if transporting the patient from one area to another.
Airborne	Place the patient in an airborne infection isolation room. Use ≥N95 respirators (or masks) while caring for patient.

74. A: Because sickle cell disease is an autosomal recessive disorder, if both parents are carriers, each of their offspring has a 25% chance of inheriting the disease. Carriers are unaffected by the disease but can pass on the defective gene to offspring.

Both parents have sickle cell trait: AS (A = normal, S = sickle cell)

	A	S
A	AA (normal)	AS (carrier)
S	AS (carrier)	SS (disease)

If both parents have the disease, then all of their children will also have the disease.

75. C: Smoking is the primary risk factor for the development of bladder cancer with smokers having triple the risk of nonsmokers. Some chemicals found in the workplace as well as arsenic in drinking water and some medications also increase the risk of bladder cancer. Caucasians are more likely to develop bladder cancer than African-Americans or Hispanics, and incidence is higher in males than females. Chronic bladder infections may also make changes in the cells, leading to cancer.

76. D: The five risk factors that the Norton scale assesses are (1) physical condition, (2) mental state, (3) activity, (4) mobility, and (5) incontinence. The Norton scale is used to assess the risk of pressure ulcers. Each item is scored on a scale of 1 to 4 with 1 being the highest risk and 4 being a normal finding. The total score can range from 5 to 20 with scores of less than 14 indicating a high risk for pressure ulcers.

77. A: If a patient who is near death from cancer repeatedly tells the nurse, "I'm going to get better and go home," the most appropriate response is "That would be wonderful." This statement is true and noncommittal and does not hold out false hope but allows the patient to hold onto personal hope. While most patients reach the stage of acceptance, some patients hold onto denial until the last possible moment. Other patients feel they must appear positive for family or friends.

78. B: A common finding with right-sided heart failure is pitting peripheral edema of the feet and ankles. Because the right side of the heart, which receives venous blood from general circulation, is impaired, blood tends to back up into the tissues. If failure is severe, the legs, back, and buttocks areas may be edematous as well. Patients may exhibit distended jugular veins and may develop ascites from portal hypertension and hepatomegaly.

79. C: When teaching a patient to do pursed-lip breathing exercises, the target inhalation to exhalation time ratio should be 1:3. That is, if inhalation lasts one second, then exhalation should last three seconds. Pursed-lip breathing is a method that helps to rid the lungs of trapped air to improve air exchange. Pursed-lip breathing involves breathing in through the nose and then breathing out slowly through pursed (circled) lips. Pursed-lip breathing is often taught to patients with chronic obstructive pulmonary disease (COPD) along with diaphragmatic breathing.

80. D: The behavioral characteristic that most places a patient at risk of suicide is when the patient's coping strategies are primarily destructive because the patient has not learned effective means of dealing with stressful situations. For example, patients who cope with stress by engaging in substance abuse are at increased risk because they are trying to ignore problems rather than dealing with them in any constructive manner.

81. A, B, and **D:** The effects that cigarette smoking have on the lungs include increased mucus production, reduction of airway diameter, and reduction of ciliary action. The cigarette smoke and nicotine cause inflammation in the upper airways, and this causes the cell walls to thicken and mucus production to increase, resulting in chronic bronchitis. Abnormal dilation of distal alveoli occurs, so instead of many tiny alveoli, these merge into large spaces with very poor air exchange. Cilia are damaged by smoking and are not able to adequately remove debris from the lungs.

82. A: When auscultating the lungs, if the nurse hears low-pitched coarse sounds that indicate secretions in the large airways, these types of breath sounds are called rhonchi. Rales (aka crackles) are fine crackling sounds (similar to the sound of rustling cellophane). Rales are frequently heard at the base of the lungs when fluid begins to accumulate. Wheezes are high-pitched whistling sounds that occur with constriction of the airways. Friction rubs are grating sounds that occur when inflamed pleural tissue rubs together.

83. C: When doing chest percussion and vibration to loosen secretions for a young adult with cystic fibrosis, the percussions should be done with cupped hands to increase vibration. Holding the hand flat can cause pain. A steady rhythm of alternating hands should be maintained while percussing different rib areas of the back and upper chest. Percussion over the spine, sternum, or lower back should be avoided. Vibration is done with the hands flat and application of pressure and shaking.

84. B: During hand-off communication, it's important to identify the patient's problems. Hand-off communication typically occurs at change of shift, during transitions of care, and during transfers. The nurse should provide only essential information, including nursing diagnoses or healthcare problems. The nurse should describe objective measures and observations and any changes in treatment or condition, establishing a clear list of priorities. The nurse should describe patient teaching or instructions as well.

85. D: If a confused older adult with no identification or information about her living situation is brought to the ED and left sitting alone in the waiting area, this type of elder mistreatment is categorized as abandonment. Patients may be left in public places or even in a home or apartment. States vary somewhat in laws regarding abandonment. For example, in some states abandonment can apply to a patient being abandoned by any usual caregiver. The laws may apply to all older adults, only to impaired older adults, and may include the disabled of any age.

86. A: When irrigating a patient's ear to remove impacted cerumen, the nurse should hold the tip of the irrigating syringe 1 cm above the ear canal so that the canal is not obscured and fluid and debris can drain out without obstruction. The patient should be in a sitting or lying position with his head turned toward the affected ear and an emesis basin placed under his ear to contain drainage. An irrigating syringe that holds approximately 50 mL of water is usually used for ear irrigations.

87. B: If a patient complains of dizziness and briefly loses consciousness after having blood drawn, the nurse should suspect that she has experienced a vasovagal reaction brought on by stress. This involuntary reaction results in a decreased heart rate and peripheral dilation, which can cause the person to feel nauseated, weak, or lightheaded and may result in fainting, especially if the patient stands. This type of loss of consciousness is referred to as situational syncope.

88. C: If a confused patient frequently climbs out of bed and walk the halls, the best approach is to apply bed/movement alarms. If the patient climbs over the side rails, it's safer to leave the side rails down because he is more likely to fall in the process of climbing over than in walking. Patients who are confused and at risk of falls should be placed within view of the nursing desk if at all possible.

89. D: With multiple myeloma, the primary initial sign or symptom of the disease is skeletal pain. The disease often goes undiagnosed in the early stages until skeletal tumors grow larger and put pressure on nerves and muscles. Eventually, the affected bones may fracture. The pain associated with multiple myeloma is most common in the back, hips, and skull. Multiple myeloma is associated with low blood counts across the board because bone marrow production is impaired.

90. A, B, and **D:** If a patient is scheduled for major abdominal surgery, preoperative instructions should include deep breathing and coughing exercises, which should be done at least every two hours after surgery. The patient should also practice incentive spirometry. In order to prevent stasis, which can lead to deep vein thrombosis (DVT), the patient should be instructed in simple leg and foot exercises, such as moving the foot up and down and in circles and doing isometric exercises. The patient should also be instructed in how to splint the incision with a pillow or hand.

91. A: If a patient wearing contact lenses splashes aftershave lotion into an eye, causing immediate tearing and burning, the first response should be to irrigate the eye with water to remove as much of the irritant as possible, then the contact lens should be removed and the eye irrigated again. The contact lens should only be removed first if immediate swelling of the eye occurs. The eye should be flushed from the inner canthus to the outer.

92. D: The type of pneumothorax that is most likely to occur if a patient's chest tube becomes obstructed is a tension pneumothorax. A tension pneumothorax is one in which pressure accumulates rapidly in the pleural space, compressing the lung on the affected side and pushing the heart and great vessels away from the affected side as well. A mediastinal shift along with severe agitation, cyanosis, dyspnea, and subcutaneous emphysema may be evident. Needle decompression may be necessary if the tube cannot be cleared immediately.

89

93. B: If an infection is spread by flying insects, such as mosquitoes, this method of transmission is vector-borne, which also includes infections caused by animals, such as dogs, or crawling insects, such as ticks. Vehicle-borne transmission occurs when an infection is spread by any substance, such as water or milk, or inanimate object (fomite), such as contaminated clothes. Direct transmission occurs through direct person-to-person contact. Airborne transmission occurs when infectious agents are spread in droplets or dust.

94. C: In the postoperative period, the patient is expected to urinate within six to eight hours, depending on the type of anesthesia and the amount of IV fluids and blood loss. The patient's bladder should be monitored carefully because she may have reduced sensation and could be at risk for a ruptured bladder if her bladder becomes overdistended. If the patient's bladder is full and the patient is unable to urinate, then catheterization may be indicated.

95. A: One-tenth of a liter is equivalent to one deciliter.

1/1000th	1/100th	1/10th	Base	×10	× 100	× 1000
milliliter	centiliter	deciliter	liter	dekaliter	hectoliter	kiloliter

96. D: If a patient has been recently diagnosed with leukemia and has been very stressed and crying, problem-focused coping strategies deal with the problem at hand (the disease) and can include attending education classes for cancer or learning independently about the disease in order to reduce stress by becoming better informed. Emotion-focused coping, on the other hand, focuses on the emotions more than the disease and can include activities to help the patient relax, such as discussing feelings, taking walks, or having massages.

97. 23 minutes: If a patient exercised for 20 minutes three days a week (total 60 minutes), 40 minutes two days a week (total 80 minutes), and 10 minutes twice a week (total 20 minutes), the patient's average exercise time per day is 23 minutes:

- 60 + 80 + 20 = 160
- 160/7 (number of days in the week) = 22.85 = 23.

98. A: If a patient is prescribed a medication that is enteric coated and it is to be administered per a patient's gastric feeding tube, the nurse should consult the physician about the medication because enteric-coated pills dissolve in the small intestine and should not be crushed for administration per gastric feeding tube. The physician may be unaware that the medication is enteric coated or may have made an error in prescribing. Pills administered per a feeding tube must be crushed completely and dissolved in liquid so that they do not block the nasogastric (NG) tube.

99. C and D: The medication orders that are written correctly include:

- 15 units Humulin R subcut. 30 minutes before meals and at bedtime.
- Vitamin D_3, 2,000 units each morning.

The orders that could be misinterpreted include the following:

- Hydrocortisone topical cream 1% applied to right arm Q.D.: This order does not indicate where on the right arm the cream is to applied, and Q.D. could be misinterpreted at QID.
- Ambien 5 mg per os at BT: Per os, which is Latin for "by mouth," is not familiar to many people, and OS can also mean "left eye." BT can be mistaken for BID.

100. B: If an older adult hospitalized after a fall has been prescribed 50 mg diphenhydramine (Benadryl) for sleep, but the nurse is concerned that this prescription is inappropriate for an older adult, the nurse should verify the prescription with the physician. Diphenhydramine is on the list of medications that should be avoided with older adults because of the risk of confusion and falls, so the nurse should express concerns about this to the physician.

101. D: The chance that a patient taking eight different medications will have a drug interaction is approximately 100%. Because of this, it's very important to accurately carry out drug reconciliation, carefully compiling a list that includes not only prescription drugs but also over-the-counter (OTC) drugs and supplements, such as vitamins and minerals. Sometimes, one drug may be given specifically to counteract the side effects of another drug (such as potassium for diuretics).

102. A: The type of angina that is associated with smoking, alcohol, and illicit stimulants is variant (Prinzmetal's) angina. For example, variant angina is a complication of cocaine use. Unlike other forms of angina, which typically occur with exertion, variant angina virtually always occurs when the patient is at rest between midnight and early morning. This type of angina tends to occur at a younger age than other types. Some medications may precipitate variant angina.

103. Two tablespoons: If a patient is prescribed 30 mL of antacid twice daily but asks how many tablespoons are approximately equal to 30 mL, the nurse should reply that two tablespoons equal about 30 mL because each tablespoon contains 15 to 16 mL. Patients should be advised to use a measuring spoon rather than a tablespoon used for dining if the patient plans to use this measurement rather than the metric one.

104. D: If an order calls for eye ointment to be applied OD, the nurse should administer the ointment to the right eye. OD is the abbreviation for the Latin term *oculus dextrus*, with *oculus* meaning *eye,* and *dextrus* meaning *right.* The left eye is indicated by OS, which stands for *oculus sinister.* Both eyes are indicated by OU, which stands for *oculus uterque.* These abbreviations, although commonly used in ophthalmology and optometry, should be avoided in prescriptions or documentation of administration because they can easily be misinterpreted.

105. B and D: Signs that are characteristic of asthma include wheezing and cough. Expiration is often prolonged because patients struggle to expel air through narrowed airways. Cough occurs as mucous production increases. Patients may feel as though they are suffocating and become very anxious and unable to speak. Sternal retraction and use of accessory muscles is often evident, and patients may become cyanotic and confused. Patients typically have tachycardia, hypertension, and profuse perspiration. With cough-variant asthma, cough is the primary indication, and wheezing may be absent altogether.

106. A: If a patient has been experiencing orthostatic hypotension, the medication that is most likely the cause is metoprolol (Inderal), which is a beta-blocker. These drugs block beta-adrenergic receptors. Thus, although the heart normally speeds up and vasoconstriction occurs when a patient changes position, the beta-blocker prevents this action so that the heart contracts with less force, and this, coupled with vasodilation, results in a drop in blood pressure when the patient changes position, such as from sitting to standing.

107. B: A patient is considered hypoxic when his pulse oximetry falls below 90%; however, because pulse oximeters can easily become dislodged, the oximeter should be repositioned and the level rechecked for low readings. If the patient's oxygenation is inadequate, he should appear in respiratory distress. The patient's vital signs and respiratory status should be assessed, and his oxygen saturation level should be reported to the physician unless this is a normal finding for the patient, such as those with advanced chronic obstructive pulmonary disease (COPD).

108. D: If a patient has episodes of fever that persist for 48 to 72 hours alternating with episodes of normal temperatures that persist for up to two weeks, the pattern of her fever is described as relapsing. This fever pattern is associated with both louse-borne relapsing fever and tick-borne relapsing fever and may be caused by one of 15 different types of spirochetes. The fever elevations occur with the release of spirochetes into the bloodstream.

109. 150 μg: If a medication is prescribed at 0.150 milligrams, the equivalent dosage in micrograms is 150 μg. Milligrams are converted to micrograms by multiplying by 1,000: 0.150 mg × 1,000 = 150 μg.

110. C and D: There are steps that a patient can take to alleviate mild sleep apnea. One of the most important is to lose weight because sleep apnea is directly associated with obesity. The patient should also sleep with her head elevated because this helps prevent collapse of the airway. Patients should avoid alcohol for three to four hours before bedtime and should also avoid taking a sleeping medication because both of these actions may increase the risk of sleep apnea.

111. A: The temperature measurement site that provides the most accurate and rapid core temperature measure is the temporal artery site. The site is easy to access, but it must be clear of hair and moisture because these can affect the results. Oral and rectal temperatures also provide fairly accurate temperatures, although both have numerous limitations. Tympanic, skin, and axillary temperatures are less reliable.

112. D: If a patient has experienced a stroke on the right side of the brain, the nurse should expect the patient to exhibit impulsivity and impaired judgment. The patient may have weakness or paralysis on the left side of the body and may experience left-sided neglect. The patient's attention span may be quite short, and he may have little concept of time. The patient's language centers remain intact, so he is able to communicate verbally.

113. B: If a patient is receiving warfarin therapy, her international normalized ratio (INR), the laboratory test done to evaluate coagulation, should generally be maintained at a range of 2.0 to 3.0. The target range may be slightly higher, 2.5 to 3.5, for those with mechanical heart valves or recurring thrombi or emboli. The INR reflects the warfarin dosage given 36 to 72 hours prior to the test. The INR is calculated based on the prothrombin time, so both test results may be reported.

114. C: If a patient's chest tube becomes dislodged, the nurse's first action should be to apply pressure to the tube insertion site. The nurse should call for assistance in order to apply a sterile dressing while the physician is notified because this is an emergent situation. If air is escaping, the dressing should not be occlusive because this can result in a tension pneumothorax. The patient should be continually monitored and assessed for hypotension, changes in breath sounds, cyanosis, and signs of tension pneumothorax.

115. A: If a patient chooses words at random, such as "The dog sun burst moving and afterwards," she is exhibiting word salad (aka schizophasia). Patients with schizophrenia or the manic phase of bipolar disorder who have disorganized thinking and speech may engage in word salad when trying to communicate. This type of disorganized thinking pattern is one of the positive symptoms of the disease. Patients may also make up words, rhyme words, or repeat the same word or phrase over and over.

116. B and D: If a nurse is to apply a transdermal nitroglycerin patch to a patient's skin, the areas that should be avoided include the abdomen and the lower arm. The abdomen should be avoided because the patch can easily be dislodged when the patient lowers undergarments to use the toilet. The lower arms and the lower legs should also be avoided because they are more likely to be exposed, increasing the risk of the patch loosening. The back is usually avoided because patches may dislodge from patient movement during sleep.

117. B: If a patient expresses concern about managing ileostomy care after discharge, the most effective reassurance is "Let's work on this together." The patient's primary concern is the inability to perform as needed, so the focus of the response should be on working toward a solution, which is itself reassuring to the patient, rather than simply providing words of reassurance, such as "Don't worry. You're smart and capable," which does little to solve the problem.

118. A and B: Characteristics that are typical of chronic illness include stable periods alternating with exacerbations during which symptoms worsen. With chronic illness, such as diabetes or arthritis, cure is rarely possible and the physical pathological changes that occur are rarely reversible. Additionally, complications tend to be frequent with chronic illness. For example, a patient with diabetes may develop hypertension, neuropathy, and renal disease. Patients with chronic illness almost always require ongoing long-term medical care.

119. 1 mL: If a patient with syphilis is to receive 600,000 units of penicillin G procaine IM and the medication is available in 2-mL vials containing 1.2 million units, the nurse should administer 1 mL of medication from the vial. The first step is to convert both measurements to either whole numbers or decimal numbers.

- Units needed/units available in dose × volume per dose = current dose.
- 600,000/1,200,000 × 2 = 1 mL.
- Or 0.6/1.2 × 2 = 1 mL.

120. C: Insulin glargine (Lantus) should not be mixed with other types of insulin in the same syringe or diluted because this may alter the pH (which is neutral) and interfere with the absorption of the insulin. Insulin glargine is a human recombinant long-acting insulin analog. It is usually administered one time daily in the morning, but it may be administered every 12 hours if necessary for glycemic control. Insulin glargine should be stored in the refrigerator but should not be frozen; however, it is stable at room temperature for 28 days.

121. A and B: Foods that are appropriate for a patient who is on the mechanically altered dysphagia diet, level 2, include meat loaf (as long as it's not too dry) and canned pears or peaches. Dry and coarse or tough meats that are difficult to chew, including fried bacon, should be avoided. Although mashed potatoes are allowed, French fried potatoes should be avoided. Soft fruits, such as bananas, and soft canned fruits, such as pears and peaches, and allowed, but fresh, frozen, and canned pineapple should be avoided.

122. B: In an adult female, the center of gravity is usually about midway between the umbilicus and symphysis pubis, whereas the center of gravity for males tends to be higher — at about the base of the sternum. In order to maintain balance, the patient's center of gravity must be over the base of support (the feet). This may mean that males and females will use their bodies somewhat differently when trying to maintain balance.

123. A: If a patient with diabetes mellitus, type 1, took insulin before lunch but ate little because of nausea and shortly thereafter became shaky, anxious, pale, diaphoretic, combative, and confused, the immediate response should be to administer quick-acting carbohydrate because these symptoms indicate an insulin reaction (hypoglycemia). Quick-acting carbohydrates include 4 to 6 ounces of a sugary drink or orange juice, 8 to 10 Life Savers, 1 tablespoon honey/syrup, 4 teaspoons jelly, or commercial dextrose.

124. C: A crisis is most likely to occur when a patient has inadequate coping strategies for a stressful event. The patient's inability to determine a course of action or a method of coping increases the stress to the point that the patient is overwhelmed. A crisis may be dispositional, may be related to life transitions, may result from trauma, may be maturational/developmental, or may reflect psychopathology. Patients may exhibit anger, aggression, withdrawal, and disorganized thinking and behavior.

125. B, C, and **D:** Common opportunistic infections associated with HIV/AIDS include tuberculosis, cytomegalovirus, and herpes zoster (shingles). Opportunistic infections are those that occur because the patient's immune system is impaired. With HIV/AIDS patients, opportunistic infections are most likely to occur when the CD4 count drops below 200 cells/mm³. There are gender differences in risks or opportunistic infections — females are more likely to develop bacterial pneumonia, and males are more likely to develop Kaposi's sarcoma.

126. D: If a patient has dysphagia and is at risk for aspiration, she should remain sitting upright for at least 30 to 60 minutes after finishing a meal. Patients should sit as upright as possible while eating and should tilt their heads slightly forward because this position makes swallowing easier. If one side of the patient's mouth is weak or paralyzed, the patient should place food and liquids on the opposite side. Thin liquids should usually be thickened.

127. B: Biot's respirations are characterized by two or three abnormally quick shallow respirations alternating with irregular periods of apnea. Biot's respirations result from injury to the pons area of the brain. This can occur with a stroke or herniation. Biot's respirations may be misclassified as Cheyne-Stokes respirations, which are similar. If Biot's respirations are evident, the patient's condition is grave.

128. A: With Raynaud's disease (intermittent digital arteriolar vasoconstriction), the patient should be advised to avoid smoking because this results in vasoconstriction, which can trigger an acute episode. Raynaud's phenomenon (red, white, and blue) occurs with vasoconstriction causing pallor (white), pallor leading to cyanosis (blue), and recovery leading to hyperemia (red). Patients must avoid cold because this triggers episodes. Primary Raynaud's disease is usually bilateral and progressive, starting with one or two digits and then spreading. The hands, feet, nose, and ears can all be affected.

129. C: The antihistamine with the highest level of sedation is diphenhydramine (Benadryl), which is an early antihistamine in the ethanolamine class and is sometimes used as a sleep aid. Later antihistamines, such as fexofenadine and loratadine, have low sedation. Antihistamines are most effective for the treatment of nasal allergies and seasonal or chronic rhinitis. Antihistamines should be avoided as sole treatment for asthmatic attacks. Drowsiness is usually the primarily adverse effect, although some users may complain of dry mouth, dysuria, and constipation.

130. B: After going to bed at night, a patient should be able to transition from awake to asleep within 10 to 20 minutes. If the patient is not asleep within 20 minutes, it's usually better to get up out of bed to do something rather than to toss and turn. People who have trouble falling asleep should be advised to avoid eating, drinking alcohol, and smoking near bedtime and to avoid caffeine. Patients should wait until they are sleepy to go to bed and should try to establish a routine bedtime.

131. C: When assisting a patient with a bed bath with soap and water, the maximum temperature of the water should be 110° to 115° F (43° to 46° C). The nurse should verify the temperature with a thermometer if possible, but at this temperature, the nurse should be able to place a finger in the water without discomfort. Because the normal body temperature is about 98.6°, water that is close to that temperature range may feel cool to the patient. Water that is too hot increases the risk of burns. The water should be changed when it begins to cool.

132. A: When applying a condom sheath to a male patient, there should be 2.5 to 5 cm distance between the tip of the glans penis and the end of the condom sheath in order to avoid irritation to the glans penis. The sheath must be applied with care with elastic adhesive applied in a spiral, nonoverlapping wrap to help secure it in place. The penis should be carefully monitored after application to ensure that circulation is not impaired.

133. B: If a patient's right leg is to be positioned in abduction (which means away from the center of the body), the best method is to place a pillow or bolster between his legs because he may forget to maintain the correct position or may move his legs during sleep. Abduction is often required following hip replacement surgery in order to reduce the risk of dislocation of the prosthesis, although this is a rare occurrence.

134. B: If a patient's blood pressure reading is typically about 135/85, her blood pressure would be categorized as prehypertension:

Category	Systolic	Diastolic
Normal	<120	<80
Prehypertension	120 to 139	80 to 89
Stage 1 hypertension	140 to 159	90 to 99
Stage 2 hypertension	≥160	≤100

135. A: Xanthine derivatives, such as theophylline, are primarily used to treat bronchoconstriction. Xanthine derivatives have been supplanted as first-line treatment of acute asthma by beta-agonists because xanthine derivatives have slower onset and more drug interactions. However, they are often used for asthma prevention and as adjunct bronchodilators for treatment of chronic bronchitis and emphysema. Adverse effects include nausea; vomiting; anorexia; reflux; as well as various cardiac abnormalities including tachycardia, extrasystole, palpitations, and ventricular dysrhythmias.

136. B: Patients who are unconscious should receive oral care routinely every two hours because the mucous membranes tend to dry out because of oxygen therapy, mouth breathing, and the inability to take oral fluids. Although lemon and glycerine swabs are sometimes available for mouth care, they may increase drying if used over a prolonged period and can damage the tooth enamel. The best solution to use is normal saline. When brushing and rinsing the patient's teeth, patients should be placed on their sides with their heads lowered so that they don't aspirate.

137. D: If a patient has experienced an overdose of oxycodone (OxyContin), the antidote is naloxone (Narcan), which can also be used for other opioid overdoses, such as morphine, heroin, methadone, butorphanol, and fentanyl. Adults are usually treated with 0.4 to 2.0 mg parenterally with doses repeated every two to three minutes as needed. If there is no response after 10 mg total has been administered, then the patient's symptoms may be caused by something other than opioids.

138. D: Although children may begin experimenting with masturbation during the phallic stage (ages 3 to 6 years), the genital stage (ages 12 and older) is the one in which masturbation and sexual relationships with peers are part of normal development according to Freud. The psychosocial stages of development include

- oral stage: ages birth to 1 year.
- anal stage: ages 1 to 3.
- phallic stage: ages 3 to 6.
- latency stage: ages 6 to 12.
- genital stage: ages 12 and older.

139. B: The phase of healing that occurs within minutes of injury and results in vasoconstriction is hemostasis. This is followed within minutes by the inflammation phase, which occurs over days 1 to 4. Phagocytosis begins and erythema, pain, and swelling may be evident. Over days 5 to 20, proliferation occurs, collagen is produced, and granulation tissue appears. The wound begins to contract. The last phase is maturation, which begins at about day 21 and continues for up to two years. During this time, scarring reduces and the tissue strengthens.

140. C: If a patient is angry with his or her physician and lashes out at the nurse, the defense mechanism that the patient is exhibiting is displacement. With displacement, the patient transfers feelings toward one target (the physician) to another (the nurse) because the second target seems less threatening to the patient. Because patients often feel intimidated by physicians, it is common for them to relieve tension by expressing anger (the most common emotion expressed in displacement) toward nursing personnel or even family members.

141. A and D: Possible indications of deep vein thrombosis (DVT) include aching, throbbing pain in the site of the thrombus (usually in the calf area), erythema (sometimes a red streak), and edema (associated with vasodilation). Some patients (but not all) may exhibit a positive Homans' sign. A positive finding is pain behind the knee when the foot is dorsiflexed. However, Homans' sign should not be used for diagnostic purposes, because its sensitivity and specificity are low.

142. D: Glasgow Coma Scale

Eye opening	4: Spontaneous. 3: To verbal stimuli. 2: To pain (not of face). 1: No response.
Verbal	5: Oriented. 4: Conversation confused, but can answer questions. 3: Uses inappropriate words. 2: Speech incomprehensible. 1: No response.
Motor	6: Moves on command. 5: Moves purposefully in response to pain. 4: Withdraws in response to pain. 3: Decorticate posturing (flexion) in response to pain. 2: Decerebrate posturing (extension) in response to pain. 1: No response.

Injuries/Conditions are classified according to the total score: 3–8, Coma; ≤8, Severe head injury; 9–12, moderate head injury; 13–15, mild head injury.

143. A: Depression is a normal response to the grief associated with bad news, such as a patient who has been diagnosed with HIV/AIDS. The patient should be encouraged to express her feelings, and the nurse should remain supportive. This stage usually passes, but if it is prolonged or if the patient becomes suicidal, then referral to a psychiatrist may be indicated. Patients may benefit from participating in a support group of other patients who are undergoing similar health problems.

144. B: The type of maladaptive grief response a patient is exhibiting if he remains fixed in the anger stage of grieving, refusing to cooperate and insulting family and healthcare providers, is distorted grieving. In this stage, the normal behaviors or feelings (such as helplessness and sadness) are exaggerated out of proportion so that the patient reacts in a volatile manner to even the smallest inconvenience. The patient often turns the anger internally and may blame himself for the problems, becoming overwhelmed with despair.

145. C: If a patient engages in moderate aerobic exercise, such as brisk walking, she should plan to exercise 150 minutes per week to meet recommended exercise guidelines for healthy adults. Patients should generally be encouraged to exercise about 30 minutes a day at least 5 days a week and to engage in strength training at least twice a week. If patients are unable to exercise for this length of time, exercising for 10 minutes three times daily provides the same benefit.

146. A: If keyboards and monitors are in each patient's room so that documentation can be done at the point of care and the monitor is mounted on the wall, when viewing the monitor, the nurse should adjust the top of the monitor so that the monitor is at or slightly below the level of the eyes. The nurse should be able to maintain the head in neutral position while viewing the monitor. Those who wear bifocals may need to have the monitor slightly lower, however, to avoid having to tip the head up.

147. D: Approximately 50% to 60% of the body weight is accounted for by water. Males tend to have a greater percentage of water than females because men usually have a greater lean body mass and fat cells contain less water than muscle tissue. For the same reason, older adults who tend to lose lean body mass have a lower percentage of water. Water is critical to the cells because it dissolves and transports nutrients, electrolytes, and waste products.

148. B: If a patient's nosebleed has stopped but the nurse notes that the patient is swallowing frequently, the nurse should suspect that blood is running down the patient's throat. If the nosebleed occurs at the back of the nasal passages, then bleeding is not always evident externally. The nurse should examine the patient's mouth and check the back of the throat. Blood is often evident in the mouth with posterior bleeding.

149. C: The movement of water between two compartments separated by a semipermeable membrane is referred to as osmosis. Solutes do not move through the membrane. The water moves from one side of the membrane to the other, from low concentration to high (the opposite of diffusion), to equalize the concentration of solutes. Osmotic pressure is the amount necessary to stop the process of osmosis and relates to the concentration of solutes in a solution.

150. A: A subcutaneous injection should be administered at a 45- to 90-degree angle, depending on the amount of subcutaneous tissue. If the nurse is able to grasp only about 2.5 cm of tissue, then a 45-degree angle should be used with a 5/8-inch needle. If the nurse can grasp 5 cm of tissue (indicating obesity), then a 90-degree angle should be used with a 1/2-inch needle, although a longer needle may be used if the patient is morbidly obese.

151. C: The normal value for potassium (K+) is 3.5 to 5.5 mEq/L. Potassium, the primary electrolyte in intracellular fluid, influences activity of the skeletal and cardiac muscles. Hypokalemia occurs at levels less than 3.5 mEq/L with the critical value at less than 2.5 mEq/L. Hyperkalemia occurs with levels greater than 5.5 mEq/L with the critical value at greater than 6.5 mEq/L.

Potassium levels depend on renal function because 80% is excreted through the kidneys and only 20% through the bowels and perspiration.

152. D: Telling a patient a personal secret is an indication that a nurse has breached a professional boundary. Liking one patient more than another is only a breach of boundary if the nurse acts on it, showing favoritism to one patient. Simple acts of kindness, such as sitting with a patient when the patient receives bad news or giving a birthday card to a long-term patient are only boundary violations if they are part of a consistent pattern of favors done for that patient and not for others.

153. B: If a hospitalized patient requests that a tribal healer participate in his treatment, the nurse should help to arrange for this to happen. Some healers use herbs or other preparations that may interfere with medical treatments, so the nurse should inquire about the type of healing procedures that will be carried out, when, and how. Every effort should be made to accommodate the patient's request and to respect the patient's traditions.

154. A: No cure is yet available for genital herpes simplex virus, type 1 or 2. Most infections are caused by type 2, but type 1 (the cause of most cold sores) can also be transmitted if people have active lesions. Palliative treatment is available with acyclovir, valacyclovir, or famciclovir. Even after the lesions (which are usually painful and blistery) clear, recurrence is possible. Genital herpes is spread through vaginal, anal, and oral sex, as well as skin-to-skin contact with infected lesions. Infants may become infected by vaginal delivery.

155. C: If a patient with obesity has begun a weight reduction program, a reasonable weekly weight loss is 1 to 2 pounds. Patients who are very obese may lose more initially, sometimes up to 5 pounds in a week, but much of this weight loss may be attributed to fluid loss, and the patient may develop unrealistic goals because of this. Patients are more likely to sustain weight loss if it occurs more slowly than if they starve themselves or exercise excessively to lose weight.

156. B: According to Maslow's hierarchy of needs, physiological needs (the need for food, water, air, body functions, sleep) must be met first because survival is dependent on these needs. Once these needs are met, then the next need is for safety and security (which includes comfort, the ability to avoid harm, and freedom from fear), followed by the need for belonging and love (giving and receiving affection, identifying with a group, interpersonal relationships). The next level of the hierarchy is the need for self-esteem/esteem of others. Maslow believed these needs must be met before a person can achieve self-actualization.

157. B and D: Early adulthood is a time of transition from adolescence into more adult roles. Early adulthood is characterized by establishment of personal/economic independence. This process may be prolonged because of a delay in entering the workforce and moving from the parents' home. This period is often one of instability and experimentation. Physical strength is usually at its peak during the decade between ages 20 and 30, after which it slowly declines. Early adulthood corresponds with Erikson's intimacy versus isolation stage.

158. A: With conscious sedation, the patient is awake but later has no memory of the procedure. Conscious sedation is often used for minor procedures, such as colonoscopies. Midazolam (Versed) is commonly used because it provides excellent amnesia. Midazolam is also sometimes administered as part of preoperative preparation when the patient must have a number of preoperative invasive procedures done, such as placement of a central venous catheter or Foley catheter, in order to reduce the patient's stress and discomfort.

159. C: After giving a patient an injection, the nurse should discard the syringe and needle intact. Attempting to recap the needle or to break or bend the needle may result in a needlestick injury and is no longer recommended. Needles should be disposed of in a special sharps hazardous waste container. These containers are often red and are made of hard plastic that needles and other sharps (blades, broken glass) cannot penetrate. The containers should be self-locking and sealable so that people cannot access them.

160. D: When carrying out CPR, the cardiac compression rate per minute should be 100. This rate is roughly equivalent to beat in the song "Staying Alive," so keeping this in mind when beginning compressions can help to establish the correct rate. Compression for adults should be at least two inches. Nonmedical rescuers now use a compression-only protocol, but medical personnel use a 30:2 compression to ventilation rate with 30 initial compressions given before ventilation is initiated.

161. A and **D:** Characteristic changes found in the gastrointestinal system of older adults include decreased production of saliva by about two-thirds, both in quantity and viscosity, interfering with breakdown of starches. Motility of the esophagus slows as does gastric emptying. Gastric mucosa atrophies, and gastric secretions become more acidic, resulting in more gastric irritation. Motility of the intestines usually remains intact (although this can be affected by medications), but there is impaired intestinal absorption of fats and nutrients.

162. A, B, and **D:** The important steps in fall prevention for older adults include encouraging patients to participate in balance and exercise programs. Patients should have annual vision and hearing examinations as well. The nurse should review patients' lists of medications to determine if any have adverse effects, such as sedation, that may contribute to falls. Although some people may have to limit activities, measures should be taken to help older adults continue with activities as much as possible. The home environment should be assessed for safety risks.

163. A: Corn is an example of a "starchy" (high-carbohydrate) vegetable. Most starchy vegetables average about 15 g of carbohydrate per 1/2 cup serving, whereas watery vegetables average about 5 g per 1/2-cup serving. Other starchy vegetables include pinto beans, lentils, peas, potatoes (white and sweet), yams, and winter squash. "Watery" vegetables include asparagus, bean sprouts, broccoli, carrots, green beans, okra, spinach and other greens, and tomatoes (technically a fruit).

164. D: If a patient tells the nurse that he has a question about the DASH diet that the nutritionist reviewed with him, the best response is "Ask me. If I don't know the answer, I'll get the information for you." The nurse should always try to answer a patient's questions promptly or offer to find the information so that the burden isn't on the patient. While it may be true that the answer is in the diet handout, there may be various reasons why the patient is unable to find the information (poor vision, low literacy, confusing text), so the nurse can help to locate and explain the information.

165. A: The routine Pap smear (recommended every three years for patients ages 21 to 65) is an example of secondary prevention. Whereas primary prevention focuses on preventing disease and tertiary prevention focuses on treating disease and preventing deterioration, the aim of secondary prevention is to identify patients with a disease in order to initiate treatment. Secondary prevention includes numerous types of screening, such as those for elevated blood pressure, tuberculosis (purified protein derivative [PPD] and chest X-rays), scoliosis, HIV infection, and diabetes.

166. B: When a patient's respiratory status must be continually monitored, the most effective method is to rely on pulse oximetry. Visual observation alone is never reliable because chest excursion may appear normal when the patient is actually in distress. Auscultation is also effective but requires moving the patient and takes more time than pulse oximetry, which can provide continuous readings. The pulse oximeter must be properly positioned to provide accurate readings.

167. C: Bioethics is the study of actions that are considered right or wrong when related to medicine, treatment, life, or death. Bioethics relates to controversial issues to which people take differing moral stands. For example, assisted suicide is a bioethical issue because some people believe it is ethical and right to assist people to die with dignity at a time of their choosing whereas others believe just as strongly that purposefully taking a life for any reason is wrong and is an act of murder.

168. D: A disinfectant that is bacteriostatic prevents the growth and reproduction of some bacteria but does not destroy bacteria as a bactericidal disinfectant does. Most of the commonly used disinfectants are bactericidal, although they may be bacteriostatic at low concentrations, so it is essential that the directions be followed exactly when disinfecting materials because if the solution is too weak or the contact time is inadequate, the desired bactericidal action may not occur.

169. C: The moral principle that decrees that the nurse provide equal care and attention to all patients is justice. This principle is usually applied to the idea that patients should have equal access to care, although the reality is that the patient's ability to pay or insurance coverage is often a prime determiner. For example, patients without insurance may not be able to have necessary surgeries, and patients who are illegal immigrants may be denied healthcare in some places.

170. B: If a nurse takes a photograph of a patient to use in a journal article without the patient's consent, this is an example of invasion of privacy. Anytime personal information or images of a patient are to be used publicly in any way, the patient must give informed consent. Invasion of privacy occurs when a nurse breaches a patient's privacy by divulging personal information to those who have no right or need to know, even if the people obtaining the information are other healthcare providers.

171. A: Items that belong to a patient should not be placed on the floor primarily because the floor is considered grossly contaminated, so anything that falls on the floor is also considered contaminated. For this reason, soiled linens or other materials should never be placed on the floor. Floors may become contaminated with an airborne organism that settles to the floor. Floors may also become contaminated by shoes or equipment. *Clostridium difficile* spores can remain viable for up to five months on floors.

172. C: If a nurse provides emergent care at the scene of an accident but the person dies from severe injuries, the nurse is protected by the state (not federal) Good Samaritan law as long as the care the nurse provided was reasonable for the situation. For example, it would be reasonable to apply pressure to stop bleeding, to carry out CPR, and to remove a patient from a burning vehicle, but it is probably unreasonable to amputate a patient's arm in order to move the patient.

173. D: If a patient has been placed in physical restraints to protect the safety of himself and others, the orders must be renewed every 4 hours for adults and 2 hours for children and adolescents, and the physical restraints may generally be maintained for a maximum of 24 consecutive hours (unless state law is more restrictive). Patients must be continually monitored while restraints are in place to ensure they are removed as soon as this can safely be done.

174. A: When removing a mask secured with two ties, the nurse should first untie the lower tie because the mask will still remain in place. Then, the nurse unties the upper tie while holding onto the ties to remove the mask. If the nurse were to remove the upper ties first, the mask could fall forward and slip down the neck because the upper ties secure the mask above the nurse's ears.

Masks should be changed if they become contaminated with fluids or secretions and if the nurse sneezes.

175. 0.84: If a female patient's waist measurement is 37 inches and her hip measurement is 44 inches, the patient's waist-to-hip ratio is 0.84: 37/44 = 0.84.

Gender	Optimal	Good	Average	Poor
Male	<0.84	0.85 to 0.89	0.90 to 0.95	≥0.95
Female	<0.75	0.75 to 0.79	0.80 to 0.86	≥0.86

176. A: If the nurse is aspirating stomach contents per an NG tube to ensure proper placement before administering a tube feeding, the pH that likely indicates gastric fluid is 4.0. Gastric fluid tends to be highly acidic, usually 4.0 or even lower. A pH reading of 7.6 is alkaline, whereas a pH of 7.38 is within the normal limits for blood (7.35 to 7.45). A pH of 7.10 is slightly acidic.

177. D: If a patient complains of rectal discomfort, abdominal distention, and flatus as well as a continuous urge to defecate and states he has passed only small amounts of liquid stool for the past three to four days, the nurse should suspect fecal impaction. The body attempts to compensate for the impaction by decreasing absorption above the impaction, and this liquid stool tends to leak around the mass of impacted stool.

178. C: If a female patient objects to a male nurse administering a vaginal suppository, the male nurse should arrange for a female nurse to administer the suppository if at all possible. Studies indicate that most female patients are accepting of male nurses, but there may be a number of reasons why female patients prefer a female nurse, including cultural standards, modesty, and a history of sexual abuse. Therefore, it's important to respect the patient's preference.

179. A: If the nurse has asked an unlicensed assistive personnel (UAP) to assist a patient with mouth care and walks by the open door to the room 30 minutes later and notes that the UAP is assisting the patient to brush his teeth, the nurse's greatest concern should be that the door is open. A patient's privacy should always be considered when providing personal care, so the curtains should be pulled around the patient's bed even if the door is closed.

180. B: During manual removal of a fecal impaction, if the patient becomes very faint with a sudden drop in blood pressure and heart rate, the most likely cause is vasovagal response. The nurse should be careful to avoid unnecessary manipulation or pressure against the rectal walls. The vasovagal response may also be caused by the pressure of the impaction alone. Manual removal of a fecal impaction should be the last resort and should be preceded by an oil retention enema to try to soften the stool and allow defecation.

181. D: Bulk-forming products, such as psyllium (Metamucil), methylcellulose (Citrucel), and polycarbophil (Fibercon) are generally the drugs of choice for chronic constipation because they increase absorption of fluid in the stool, helping to increase mass, soften stool, and stimulate peristalsis. Bulk-forming products have few adverse effects and are less irritating to the intestines than other preparations. However, if fluid intake is inadequate, bulk formers can cause obstruction, so they should be avoided with patients who are dehydrated or on fluid restriction.

182. B: If a patient's hand is swelling and a ring is beginning to impair circulation, the first method to use in attempting to remove the ring is elevating and soaking the hand in cool water for about five minutes to try to reduce edema and then applying lubricant such as dishwashing soap or lubricant jelly liberally about and under the ring. It's important to avoid damaging the tissue. If this method is ineffective, then the string wrap method may be tried before cutting the ring with a circular saw, which should be the last resort unless the risk of gangrene is severe.

183. A: Following a vasectomy, the comment by the patient that indicates a need for education is "I know that sterility is almost immediate after vasectomy." In fact, sterility can take more than 8 weeks to attain. Patients should have a postvasectomy semen analysis after 8 to 16 weeks (physicians vary in the timeframe). Patients should avoid ejaculation for one week and then should use alternate means of contraception until occlusion of the vas is confirmed through testing.

184. C: Patients with cognitive impairment and the inability to verbalize pain may appear tense and frightened and exhibit increased combativeness when they have pain. Respirations may become more rapid and labored. Patients may remain silent and withdrawn or begin to moan or cry out, especially as pain increases. Patients in pain often are very difficult to console or distract. The Pain Assessment IN Advanced Dementia (PAINAD) tool is helpful when assessing pain in patients with cognitive impairment and evaluates breathing, negative vocalization, facial expression, body language, and consolability.

Thank You

We at Mometrix would like to extend our heartfelt thanks to you, our friend and patron, for allowing us to play a part in your journey. It is a privilege to serve people from all walks of life who are unified in their commitment to building the best future they can for themselves.

The preparation you devote to these important testing milestones may be the most valuable educational opportunity you have for making a real difference in your life. We encourage you to put your heart into it—that feeling of succeeding, overcoming, and yes, conquering will be well worth the hours you've invested.

We want to hear your story, your struggles and your successes, and if you see any opportunities for us to improve our materials so we can help others even more effectively in the future, please share that with us as well. **The team at Mometrix would be absolutely thrilled to hear from you!** So please, send us an email (support@mometrix.com) and let's stay in touch.

If you feel as though you need additional help, please check out the other resources we offer:

Study Guide: http://MometrixStudyGuides.com/NursingACE

Flashcards: http://MometrixFlashcards.com/NursingACE